Baby Greens

Baby Greens

A Live-food Approach for Children of All Ages

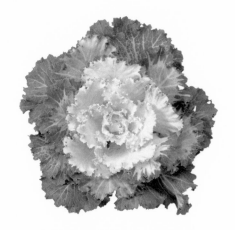

Michaela Lynn ✦ Michael Chrisemer

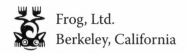
Frog, Ltd.
Berkeley, California

Published by Frog, Ltd.

Frog, Ltd. books are distributed by
North Atlantic Books
P.O. Box 12327
Berkeley, California 94712

Cover design by Paula Morrison
Book design by Jan Camp
Printed in the United States of America

Baby Greens is sponsored by the Society for the Study of Native Arts and Sciences, a nonprofit educational corporation whose goals are to develop an educational and cross-cultural perspective linking various scientific, social, and artistic fields; to nurture a holistic view of arts, sciences, humanities, and healing; and to publish and distribute literature on the relationship of mind, body, and nature.

North Atlantic Books' publications are available through most bookstores. For further information, call 800-733-3000 or visit our website at www.northatlanticbooks.com.

ISBN 13: 978-1-58394-137-9

Library of Congress Cataloging-in-Publication Data

Lynn, Michaela, 1975–
    Baby greens: a live-food approach for children of all ages / by Michaela Lynn
and Michael Chrisemer ; preface by Gabriel Cousens.
        p. cm.
    Includes bibliographical references.
    ISBN 1-58394-137-1 (pbk.)
    1. Children—Nutrition. 2. Infants—Nutrition. 3. Natural foods. 4. Raw food diet.
5. Bioenergetics. I. Chrisemer, Michael, 1952– II. Title.
    RJ206.L96 2005
    649'.3—dc22

                                                                    2005016804

2 3 4 5 6 7 8 9 United 14 13 12 11 10 09 08

❧ Table of Contents

❧ Note of Gratitude

Special thanks to Lars Marshall for your many talents: computer assistance, enthusiasm, grace, humor, and generosity (to name a few). A big thanks to the Patagonia Public Library, its volunteers, and to Anne Sager for never kicking me off the computers. Thank you Jeffrey Cooper, Will Hadley, and to Lars for your "technical difficulty" rescues.

We give gratitude for all whose visionary work spreads the joy of living foods.

Dedicated of course to the kiddies and to the living child in everyone here, in the days between.

Hearts of summer held in trust, still tender, young, and green,
Left on shelves collecting dust, not knowing what they mean,
Valentines of flesh and blood, as soft as velveteen,
Hoping love will not forsake the days that lie between.

— Robert Hunter

❧ Preface

Baby Greens by Michaela Lynn and Michael Chrisemer is a delightful, heartfelt, educational primer and support system for parents. It has imaginative, fun-filled, easy recipes, useful resources, and practical parent-child activities to potentiate the live-food way of life. It represents, for me, the birth of a seed planted at the Tree of Life—one of much needed support for parents, babies, and older children on the live-food path and natural-foods lifestyle.

The essential question that parents ask when they get this information is: Can a live-food diet be safe for my child? This fundamental question needs to be answered both publicly and privately. The Tree of Life Foundation study of the effect of the live-food diet on pre-adolescent children and babies, by measuring height and weight, answers that question in a way that helps parents confidently read this book. The results of this study completely support live-food parents, their way of being, and their success in bringing children into a new paradigm and quality of life. The Tree of Life study, which included twenty children, showed that the heights of 90% of the live-food children were in the 25th percentile or higher. The weights of 75% of the live-food children were in the 25th percentile or higher. We found that the heights of 60% of the live-food children were in the top 25th percentile or higher, and the weights of 25% of the live-food children were in the top 25th percentile or higher. In other words, about 80% of the live-food children were between the lowest 10% and highest 10% of the scale. Two-thirds of these live-food children were considered average or above average in height and weight. Parents can proceed confidently knowing that two-thirds of the live-food children in the

Tree of Life Foundation research study were average or above average, and all children were above the lowest 10th percentile in height and weight as provided by the National Center for Chronic Disease Prevention. A properly followed live-food diet for mother and child is not only totally safe, but incredibly beneficial.

With this very important piece of information in hand, parents, following the pregnancy and post-pregnancy nutrition for mothers and children, can expect to have very healthy children, as measured by height and weight.

Once we are clear that the live-food diet is perfectly safe, we can read this wonderful little book with a sense of relief and appreciation for the heartfelt, mother-centered point of view in which it was written. This book is a delightful bridge into an optimal quality of life that is healing for ourselves, our children, and the whole living planet.

I give thanks to Michaela and Michael for their wonderful contribution to the health and support of all families, particularly live-food families. I consider *Baby Greens* a must read for all, especially live-food, parents.

— Gabriel Cousens, M.D., M.D. (H), Dip. in Ayurveda
and director of the Tree of Life Foundation, Patagonia, AZ

❧ Foreword
The Raw-Foods-Dominant Diet

Anyone attempting to learn about nutrition can easily become confused by contradictions, controversy, and the many different approaches. New parents and parents-to-be are, additionally, often apprehensive about how best to provide nutrition that is as nurturing and complete—once feeding with solid food begins—as breast-feeding was before. Add to this the fear of toxins in the food chain, persistent misinformation touting the inadequacy of a vegetarian-based diet, antiquated information guiding mainstream nutrition generally, and the convoluted picture is complete.

Our purpose in writing *Baby Greens* is to provide a nutritional primer of informative support, recipes, resources, and activities to help you and your children begin to resolve these issues and either start a living-foods lifestyle or deepen the one you already practice. By "informative support" we mean the ABCs of bioenergetic nutrition. Bioenergetic nutrition simply means consideration of the much more subtle, or energetic, qualities as well as the solid, physical presence of both foods and the human organism. We feel that an elementary grounding in how nutrition and health are viewed bioenergetically is essential for building the confidence that is so helpful in maintaining a doubt-free transition from cooked and processed foods to your own style of a raw-foods-dominant diet. Since the cooking of food renders it largely devoid of enzymes, life force, and many nutrients, these foods require energy from us to digest and assimilate. Living, raw foods, on the other hand, add far more energy than they take away for digestion.

It is important, therefore, to create meals in which raw or uncooked foods dominate. A fifty-fifty mix is a minimum recommendation of where to begin. An important distinction to make is that not all raw foods are necessarily living foods. Raw nuts and seeds, for example, need to be soaked in order to once again become truly living foods. From this point they can sprout, or be processed otherwise for use in raw-foods-dominant recipes. Produce that was a living food after harvest might not continue to be so if too much time passes. Fresh produce in the sense of locally grown and less than a few days old is one ideal way to go. Fresh, same-day garden produce is obviously then the best choice, if available, for fully living food.

Whatever degree or style of natural foods diet is your practice, interacting with your child's enjoyment of these living foods and fostering his/her intuitive fulfillment of unique nutritional needs can become a mirror—a wonderfully intrinsic encouragement to your own process of returning to a more balanced relationship with food, for children learn by what we do and what we say. When they can witness us living new modes of life, they can easily follow in natural synchronicity. Because of their small physical size, babies and young children are so much more susceptible than adults to the thousands of toxins in the environment and the commercial food supply today. Elimination of food-related toxins from our children's diets is a powerful boost to all levels of their health. You could say it is an investment, an insurance of incomparable value. The growing and learning that children are here to do is far freer to progress when a living-foods-dominant diet underlies the living innocence of non-possessive, non-authoritarian parenting.

We have tried to write from a fully contemporary, naturopathic point of view—a view too often marginalized, lost, or omitted from mainstream thought and nutritional practice. We offer an effective framework that will help provide the confidence and knowledge necessary to move beyond the fear, doubt, misinformation, and controversy surrounding child nutrition, and allow the innate order of living foods and the naturopathic point of view to be your guides. We hope the support and insight offered here will ease the transition, acting as a bridge toward living nutrition and away from the standard dietary wasteland of over-processed, dead, and contaminated fare. The short, medium, and long-term rewards of this transition are priceless for you and your child. The costs of reliance on the standard American diet are tragically apparent for anyone with eyes to see.

Much of the confusion and controversy in nutrition today still originates from one source: the loss of the concept of our foods and the soil from which they grow as a living system. Even if we have the concept intellectually, we might still be disconnected from its meanings and thus disconnected from the active understanding that we achieve vibrant health by maintaining an intimate connection to the living earth through consumption of living foods.

In matters of healthcare a similar situation exists: we've become doubtful about our innate abilities to heal. When we rediscover living, non-toxic nutrition as an irreplaceable part of our daily therapy, namely our daily regeneration, recreation, and relaxation, then we can truly go further. Nutrition need not remain a missing link to the larger reality of authentic wellness.

In the midst of the confusion surrounding child nutrition, few have had the opportunity to visualize clearly the incredible potential for vibrant health and depth of wellness, far beyond current norms, that exists for children who are raised with living foods. This is especially important in a time when toxic interferences throughout the environment demand that we establish a foundation of genuine health quickly for our kids, by the most efficient and effective means possible. An impressive accumulation of research says conclusively that a living-foods-dominant diet is a major component of such efficient and effective means.* We hope this book will help unlock a door or two and allow you to step back and say something like, "Hmmm, this works!"

---

*See "Putting It All Together: Ideas and Guidance for the Individual Health Plan," page 31.

Take a look around at the kids in your schools and the growing statistics. There are more cases of childhood obesity, allergies, and illnesses. More children are on Ritalin and other dangerous drugs including vaccines than ever before. It is the authors' belief that much of the behavioral chaos and learning inability so common in many homes and in many public schools could be significantly cleared if standard food service meals were replaced with living-foods-dominant meals. Of course, a living curriculum at home and/or in school would not hurt either.

The false disease labels of Attention Deficit Disorder (ADD) and Attention Deficit Hyperactivity Disorder (ADHD) created by the medical cartel to "help" even the youngest children (and these days, maybe even their parents) are, in nearly all cases, symptomatic pictures of nutritional deficiency not diseases in need of toxic "cures." Indeed, a crucial difference between the naturopathic and mainstream medical allopathic models is that pure naturopathy generally places all manner of illness not in categories of disease but under the more causal reality of nutrition. Nutrition in this broadest and deepest sense is the vast arena of not only food but also detoxification, hydration, healing, and regeneration of the whole person, in other words, of all that nourishes.

We are still free to exchange confusion and controversy for our rightful, innate clarity anytime. As we do, our children will be the beneficiaries of this one simple yet profound shift. May we all continue the process.

> — Michael Chrisemer
> Patagonia, AZ
> January 2003

❧ Introduction
Conception of Baby Greens

I hadn't questioned the established tradition of boiling, baking, frying, and sautéing until I read *Why Suffer*, the autobiography of Anne Wigmore. Charmed by her tales of a childhood kinship with nature, I read on as she told of the whole new world of the city and the perils of disease that met her there. In awe I continued as young Anne recovered from terminal gangrene, a solitary struggle for life and limb, and was rescued by none other than earth's miracle workers: flowers, grass, sunshine, water, and a puppy. Further inspired by her later discoveries, I began to grasp for the first time a concept of living nutrition. Like most everyone else whose everyday sustenance has always been cooked, the inherent life of my food was more or less unknown to me. In its natural simplicity the idea of eating raw food rang true, but making a radical change in my lifestyle was more difficult to swallow.

My curiosity piqued, I started taking baby steps. I grew wheat grass and sprouts, dusted off my juice extractor, and began to experiment with raw-food preparation. As my repertoire of recipes began to grow, I noticed that the more alive my food became, the more alive I felt. After years of having been failed by dozens of skin products, fistfuls of vitamin supplements, and a prescription for a drug that is known to cause birth defects (in children of women who take it while pregnant), the acne-plagued complexion I had been suffering since my adolescence was slowly beginning to clear. Healing continued to snowball as I was introduced to spinal therapy at a Network Spinal Analysis clinic, and I gained, through this, a new understanding of the relationship between my habits of thought and their expressions in the physical body. Past traumas and bottled emotions found new release, and greater self-acceptance began to unfold. Children were no longer inquiring as to my "chicken pox." To the contrary, people began to tell me that I was "glowing"—"radiant" even. They wanted to know what I was doing differently!

Having married and moved to the Southwest (from the Midwestern U.S.), I started working for the Tree of Life Rejuvenation Center in Patagonia, AZ. In this living-foods-retreat setting I gained more insight for my dietary transitioning. Talking with others making similar changes, I compared notes on what had worked for us, and what had not. Raw-food chefs and apprentices also served up fresh ideas and inspiration for my own new culinary dabbling. My work, which involved taking dictations for the writings of Dr. Gabriel Cousens (author of *Conscious Eating* and *Spiritual Nutrition*), also became a generous helping of food for thought.

It wasn't long after I began my work at Tree of Life that Michael and I discovered we were going to have a baby! As we prepared for her arrival, resources in natural childbirth fell serendipitously into place. When the time approached to introduce little Quinn to her first solid foods, however, the more that I researched, the less I seemed to find on living nutrition for young children. From leading authorities on infant care I gleaned general insights such as when she might be ready for initial samplings and which foods can pose potential hazards or sensitivities; but aside from breast milk, I found their suggested diets to be almost exclusively made up of cooked foods (and in the case of commercial baby foods heated up to twelve times!).

Within the arena of raw-nutrition I found that despite its growing interest, with health testimonials by the thousands, precious little has been written on the integration of these ideas into the lives of our children. I found this to be especially true when addressing the specific needs of infants and toddlers.

One reason for this information gap seems to be the increasingly controversial nature of nutrition in general. The more that is discovered of our food elements and their varied effects on the body, the more theories, fads, and diets seem to follow. Even with the basic, common-sense approach of eating food in its raw and natural state, one need not look far to find opposing viewpoints. "Take carrots, for example," said a man I had spoken to for advice. "One person says they're the best thing for you, another claims they're the worst, and both have the research to prove it." With this endless range of conflicting expertise it is not hard to imagine how some parents have been intimidated by the subject.

In addition to the controversy, there is significant motivation to turn a blind eye to the discoveries made in living nutrition. Although we are seekers of health and wellness as an over-consuming nation, we are very attached (if not addicted) to the way that we eat; and in my experience, change to our way of life is seldom met without some resistance. Having even more profound of an influence on the nutritional information we read are perhaps the financial investments at stake. From meat and dairy to pharmaceutical products, many corporate structures' security depends on our eating habits and dietary beliefs remaining loyal to them.

Nutrition's stormy debate with its host of divided interests becomes all the more emotionally charged when it comes to feeding our children. As parents we seek what is best for their developing bodies, but as we look to the experts for their counsel, we often find ourselves blown and tossed about by the rapidly shifting winds of opinion. It was after one such series of failed fact-finding missions that I stumbled upon an epiphany. I recognized within myself more than the desire to be well informed. I saw also the presence of fear. I hadn't found a final authority on living foods for my baby and was becoming increasingly uneasy. Revisited by my previous lessons with authority, I began to see my social conditioning to look outside myself for the final word on what is best for my own family. In my own reflection, I saw a society that urges unquestioned allegiance to leadership at the expense of individuals not recognizing their own distinct voices of discernment, intuition, and instinct. And so my final authority emerged. With the grace not to banish conventional wisdom altogether, my innate intelligence took throne. I felt a new confidence to care for my young, an ability that although hidden from me had been underlying all along.

It was after this revelation, interestingly, that more information began to find its way to me. It didn't come in the form of an entire book devoted to the subject of living foods for little ones, as I had so fervently sought out. Instead it arrived in bits and pieces, trickling in steadily from a diverse range of sources. *Baby Greens* has become the book I've been looking for and was written in the spirit of self-trust and empowerment.

The lack of resources on living nutrition for children has moved Michael and me profoundly to write this book, but rather than to stake claim of unique authority on the subject, we hope to hold up a light to the instinctive wisdom within each reader and within each reader's child. In addition, it is not our intention to promote rigid dietary perfectionism or to set one standard for all families to measure against. Observing many attitudes often surrounding food (including my own), I have come to believe that a balanced diet involves more than simply that which enters our mouths, and this strike of balance may appear fairly different from one household to another. This book aims to serve the needs of a variety of nutritional lifestyles. We have sought to help fill a gap of information and form a bridge between the standard American animal-based diet and a whole-and-living-plant-based lifestyle. To help with dietary transitions we have included some cooked food ingredients in a portion of the recipes. The "Family Activities" section for children reflects what we've learned as parents and in our professional relationships with children—that is: The desire to learn and to grow is inherent, and it will naturally thrive in an environment that nurtures children's innate joy and autonomy. In the recipes you will also see an element of play, for it is our final hope in writing this book to bring more life into your mealtime together and laughter into your kitchen.

    — Michaela Lynn
    Patagonia, AZ
    February 16, 2003

Part I

Collected Essays on Health and Bioenergetic Nutrition

by Michael Chrisemer, N.C.

Mind-Set: Recognitions and Adaptations

Human beings are remarkably adaptive. We rebuild and regenerate all the time. However, the existing standard American paradigm of nutrition is woefully inadequate for assisting development of the reality into which we are capable of evolving. Nutrition is obviously about more than physical food groups. Of equal and ultimately more importance are the subtle properties of living foods. When we follow the traditional norms of cooked and processed foods, we lose access to these subtle properties and in the process one very critical aspect of our potential for other modes of growth. The main action of subtle nutritional processes goes on at other, largely invisible, levels. For instance, what we witness with digestion and metabolism is only the tip of the iceberg in this largely invisible human being. Nutrition is, however, the most readily accessible and influential place for us to begin to set in order our individual, internal nutritional ecology.

Becoming a vegetarian or even a vegan is one thing. As different and as healthful as these nutritional lifestyles are compared to the standard American diet, so too, the organic, raw-food, vegan lifestyle appears to be as dramatically different when compared to standard cooked-food vegetarianism. Many would argue that in fact it is the raw-food component of the standard vegetarian diet that makes the most difference for health and wellness. New understanding of the critical need to individualize the diet to more closely match one's constitutional biochemical individuality is beginning to quietly revolutionize nutrition. It is now possible to move beyond the one-size-fits-all dietary prescriptions, food pyramids, and calorie counting schemes and first determine one's real nutritional needs. One can then experiment with embodying these needs in a more-correct-for-your-metabolism-ratio of protein, carbohydrate, and fat that will optimize pH balance, energy, and ultimately one's whole health picture.

Whatever degree of raw foods you are able to incorporate into your child's diet to begin with is a good thing! A fifty-fifty mix of raw to cooked food on a meal-for-meal basis makes a very noticeable difference for a lot of people. Try this with your child and see where the child's and your balance lie. As mentioned in the foreword, information is not enough. A change in what food means to us is necessary, thus new and more active understandings can occur.

For many reasons society is still cognitively stuck in an old mind-set where nutrition is concerned. In this case new information is deemed anathema. When this is so, self-built blocks prevent information from ever reaching the level of understanding. Good and valid information full of meanings is out there, but much of it in this living-foods arena has yet to penetrate to the level of understanding for much of society. We all need to move forward into higher, more-refined modes of nutritional practice while simultaneously acknowledging that society might take a while to learn the same things.

Being aware of both the ongoing visible and invisible processes in ourselves and our children—that have potentials to subtly lead us either to higher levels or to places of stagnation and probable ill-health—is a powerful tool for discovering all manner of blockages and transforming them. Participating with our children in a raw-foods-dominant diet and watching them thrive on it—without meat, without dairy, without processed foods, and without all the sundry accoutrements of the standard American diet—is one of the most effective means we have in creating a high probability for our children to be successful at health building. Children have the capacity to bring all kinds of abilities into their awareness if only we give them opportunities to exercise in the direction of these abilities. An effective plan for wellness involves presenting the young child with opportunities to learn how to make use of living foods, how to release tension from the spine and nervous system, and how to realize the "higher mind." Assisting your child with these discoveries is the reason for being for *Baby Greens*—we wish you every good success in your experience of wholeness.

Reestablishing the Whole Picture

Mainstream, nutritional science has analyzed and dissected the intricacies of the human body's grosser metabolic and nutritional processes. Foods have also been exhaustively taken apart and many of their elements identified. However, in terms of putting things back together again to form a more complete whole picture, one that truly enlivens understanding via the natural mind, we are left on our own.

For all its technological brilliance, mainstream science is cognitively blinded by a mind-set that is inadequate to the task of reestablishing the whole picture of child nutrition in a way that many of us would like. Bioenergetic nutritional science, on the other hand, has a dramatically different methodology for analyzing and understanding a much bigger picture of both the obvious and more-subtle metabolic processes. The mainstream, materialistic approach views food as only material, like protein, carbohydrates, fats, etc. Energy is measured only in caloric content. In contrast to bioenergetic nutrition, this materialistic or mechanistic view does not take into account that we are multidimensional beings, capable of absorbing and utilizing other, more-subtle energies that also nourish and support life processes.

As mentioned earlier, the source of much confusion and controversy in nutrition is the loss of the concept of our foods growing in a living system of soil. When you no longer know your food to be alive, conventional wisdom says to salt, skin, dilute, cook, can, adulterate, and/or irradiate the food into dead stuff—the stuff of which childhood health problems are made. Conversely, when we make the initial connection of understanding food as inherently alive, many previous questions about child nutrition are naturally resolved. A realization dawns of just how fitting the raw-foods-dominant diet is for young peoples' nutritional needs. So, why eat raw foods as a major component of any diet?

Enzymes, Digestion, the Pancreas, and the Subtle Terrain

If perpetuation of the standard American diet hinges on the loss of knowledge of living foods, then so does the whole convoluted picture of dietary confusion and ill health that is the norm, sadly, for those who adhere to the heavily processed, standard American diet. To easily understand why raw foods can rebalance the whole organism, thus restoring optimal health, we can focus on one key area: how digestion ideally works.

By far the largest part of digestion is accomplished by enzymes. Every raw food has naturally occurring enzymes, enough to digest that particular food. An apple, for instance, contains the right amount of enzymes needed for your body to digest it. Enzymes are destroyed by heat. Beginning at a temperature of 105°F the enzyme content of food is rapidly lost. Cooking foods can also kill other nutrients, render natural oils indigestible, produce toxic chemical by-products, and destroy the life-force—the Subtle Organizing Energy Fields (SOEFs)—present in living foods.

So then, how do we digest foods whose enzymes and other elements have been destroyed? We must draw on the body's reserves of digestive and other enzymes. As mentioned before, we must often use more energy than we get to attempt to digest cooked foods. Digestive enzymes are produced by the pancreas and only function in an alkaline environment. The pancreas also secretes sodium bicarbonate to create this alkaline environment for the acidic contents of the stomach as they enter the small intestine for further digestion.

Pancreatic burnout is present to a considerable degree in 90% of people tested. Eating large, cooked meals stresses the pancreatic output of enzymes and sodium bicarbonate. The pancreas is also highly sensitive to toxins such as pesticides, caffeine, alcohol, and the thousands of potentially toxic chemicals in our drinking water. This is true whether you have food sensitivity issues or can generally do well on any good variety of foods. Organically grown, raw, living foods reduce the depletion of the body's enzyme reserves. What can typically happen when enzyme production cannot keep up with processed food intake? Absorption of partially digested proteins and other toxic by-products of cooking into the bloodstream can cause allergic reactions and further intoxication of the immune system. Remember, our immune system identifies and eliminates that which is not us. Foreign or undigested substances in our blood cause an immune reaction called leucocytosis. This is a rapid production of large numbers of white blood cells immediately following ingestion of cooked foods, especially animal products. Unlike our muscles, our immune system does not strengthen the more it is exercised; it slowly weakens, especially when the response to deal with foreign matter in the blood is evoked several times daily! By adopting a raw-foods-dominant diet you can dramatically reduce or even avoid this whole burdensome process.

Just as the breakdown of digestion produced by a toxic, highly refined, and overcooked diet creates a ripple effect through metabolic blockage, chronic energy drain, toxic bioaccumulation, and immune over-stimulation that eventually affects physical, emotional, and other levels of well-being, so the introduction of organically grown, raw, living foods is a critical foundational support for the reversal of these conditions and initiating the restoration of balance.

Organically grown, raw, living foods provide the highest profile of truly usable elements while naturally conserving the digestive and immune functions. Raw foods naturally tend to keep the body alkaline, another key consideration in health building. Raw foods provide the broadest support to remedy multiple food sensitivities and allergies, although in these cases further individual diet testing and tailoring is wise.

Raw foods are naturally free of all the toxins that better nutritionists routinely target for elimination from the diet, no matter what. These toxic elements are: food additives of all kinds; refined flour and sugar; milk; coffee and black tea; alcohol; chocolate; animal products; and MSG, to name the worst and obvious few. To our negation of what society has for so long taken for granted as being perfectly fine—namely consumption of refined and processed foods—we must add many forms of cooked food. This is the conceptual leap that can be more easily taken when some idea of the subtlety of nutritional homeostasis, or balance, is grasped.

Higher profiles of useable elements, alkalinizing effects on the body, energy gain rather than loss, and the non-toxic nature of raw foods provide protection against the many possible internal imbalances that can become causal factors in ill-health. The concept of the biological terrain, or internal environment in which organs operate, as intimately linked to health through nutritional practices has been refined into an art and a science. Nutritional deficiencies, toxic levels in various organs, and the associated metabolic blockages and imbalances need, for the most part, never arise in children who maintain a balanced and nutritively complete terrain through a raw-foods-dominant diet.*

---

*See http://www.terrainmed.com for an overview of terrain testing.

Nutritional Individuality:
Metabolic Individuality, Brain Response,
Intuitive Eating, and Recipe Rotation

The concept of nutritional individuality is key to understanding why any given diet might or might not work well. The various dietary systems, prescriptions, or "one-size-fits-all" approaches are very limiting—first, because many diets are not primarily composed of organically grown, living foods; second, because we all have unique nutritional needs based, in some part, on our genetic inheritance. In reality, one size can never possibly work for all. Genetic inheritance can be translated as: How are my various metabolic systems predisposing me to need certain foods rather than others? It could also translate as: How does this "metabolic individuality" of mine produce, for instance, an alkaline response from certain food when my son gets an acid result from the same food?

Remember that the body is constantly producing acidity via its various functions such as regeneration of tissues, digestion, and assimilation of food. In addition to the acidic by-products of metabolism, exercise and negative thinking also produce acids in the body. It is critical that we help the body maintain its proper blood pH. The range here is strictly a very narrow one—between 7.3 and 7.5, which is slightly alkaline, for optimal health to flourish. Why do the various prescription diets work for some people, but not for others? What the latest research says is truly revolutionary in its implications. Knowing one's individual metabolic tendencies can truly make a huge difference for wellness. The more choices we have, the more subtle our health and wellness can become. The individualized, raw-foods-dominant diet: Get to know it for yourself; you'll like it!

Research by Williams, Wolcott, Cousens, and others strongly suggests that food is not the sole determinant of acid or alkaline effects in the body. It is, rather, the dominant regulatory or metabolic system of the individual that really determines whether specific nutrients including vitamins and minerals will produce an acid or an alkaline result in the body. There is, within the dominant metabolic system of a given individual, also a range of tendency to constitutionally be more acidic or more alkaline.

The oxidative system, for example, appears to be dominant in approximately 50% of the population. The oxidation process is all about energy production in the body. A slow oxidizer produces energy from glucose too slowly. A fast oxidizer has a glycolysis cycle that works too quickly. Balanced oxidation can be achieved through diet and lifestyle changes. However, if one is oxidative dominant, then fruits and vegetables will tend to acidify the blood while fats and proteins will move the blood toward alkalinity. In addition, as mentioned, there is also a range of possible constitutional tendency between slow and fast oxidation at work here. The slow oxidizer, for example, constitutionally tends toward the alkaline. The fast oxidizer tends toward acid. So, if one is an oxidative-dominant, slow oxidizer, then even though the oxidative-system dominance will tend to produce an acid result from fruits and vegetables, the constitutional tendency of the slow oxidizer is toward alkalinity—thus fruits and vegetables reacting in an acidifying way would tend to balance this natural tendency toward alkalinity. In an oxidative-dominant, fast oxidizer, however, the constitutional tendency toward acidity would be exaggerated by a high-carb diet.

The Autonomic Nervous System (ANS) is also dominant in roughly half of the population. If one is ANS-dominant, fruits and vegetables alkalinize the blood, whereas fats and proteins acidify it. The range of constitutional tendency here is between sympathetic and parasympathetic dominance. A sympathetic-dominant person tends, constitutionally, toward acidic blood. Parasympathetic dominance tends toward alkaline blood. So, in the ANS/sympathetic-dominant person the constitutional tendency toward acidity will be balanced by the ANS-dominant production of an alkaline reaction from fruits and vegetables. In the ANS/parasympathetic-dominant person the parasympathetic alkaline constitutional tendency would be further exaggerated by the ANS production of an alkaline reaction from fruits and vegetables. This is a profound departure from the typical teachings on the relationship between diet and the acid/base balance in the body.

For those inclined to be their own scientists and apply this concept to themselves, pH-testing paper, available at drugstores, allows one to do simple pH testing of the urine. The recommended method is to collect urine samples in the same container, over the course of an entire 24-hour period, beginning with the second urine of the morning and ending with the first urine the next morning. Stir and test the whole mix the following morning (dip a piece of the pH paper in the urine). This will tell you the average effect that your diet is having on pH and will allow you to modify the diet and see the effects of these modifications on pH. This can produce insight toward understanding which mix of foods (carbohydrates, proteins, and fats) best balances the pH for you.

It is easy to understand why the two oxidative types mentioned above require a different ratio of protein, carbohydrate, and fat for the achievement of optimal health. The fast oxidizer tends to be too acidic and does best on a high protein (50%), low carbohydrate (30%), and moderate fat (20%) diet. As you might guess, balanced oxidizers are more the norm, and they tend toward a balanced pH and do well on a diet of moderate protein (40%), moderate carbohydrate (40%), and moderate fat (20%). For most people the percentage of protein or carbohydrate in their diet doesn't seem to be too critical. They will do fine if they eat a wide variety of organically grown foods prepared in their raw, living state. If, however, you or your child is among a smaller but significant number (and growing) of people who are food sensitive, allergic, and thus perhaps metabolically imbalanced, this approach will not work. It is important to note that when your diet is at least 50–75% raw food on a consistent and meal-for-meal basis, then many food sensitivities and allergies can be more easily and quickly healed, assuming that the offending foods are eliminated and, if worthy, rotated back into the diet when the imbalance can be cleared. Theorizing that complex metabolic imbalances and their myriad concomitant health problems can, eventually, be balanced by the raw-foods-dominant diet seems like high-order common sense. Still, testing and tailoring of the diet when the problems don't respond is wise. It is still obviously theory as to whether or not children who are raised "raw" will be inherently less susceptible to metabolic dominance of one type or another.

How plastic or how changeable is one's genetic inheritance? It is well known, for example, that a slow-oxidizing person can convert to faster oxidation by exercising approximately twenty minutes twice a day for a minimum of six months. Conversely, a fast oxidizer will often convert to a slower oxidizer if this person remains sedentary for more than a couple of years. And how does chronic fight-or-flight tension, locked up in the spine and nervous system, affect metabolic-dominance issues? Isn't a general metabolic balance the natural product of the most natural diet—the raw-foods diet? In any case, basic terrain testing is extremely economic, paints a very accurate picture of nutritional/metabolic disturbances, and is recommended for everyone—especially if you or your child has become food sensitive, allergic, or deficient, or if your metabolic dominance is off the norm.

Many food sensitivities and allergies develop because a particular food is eaten too frequently. For example, if you feed your baby almonds most days, beware, for you could be creating food sensitivity. If eating high-quality, raw almonds can cause a food sensitivity, imagine what can result when processed or pesticide-laden foods are used. Quality of food is critical; however, quantity and frequency also carry critical influence—especially when we take into account possible underlying, individual, metabolic influences. We suggest rotating the recipes with regard to ingredients. The recipe rotation concept is based on preparing meals from one large set of foods for two to three weeks and then rotating to another set of foods for the same period. We feel that this is a great way for children to avoid over-exposure to any one group of foods. It could theoretically work to minimize the evocation of problems associated with incompatibility of foods due to metabolic-type issues. The recipe rotation can be as informal or as finely tuned as your needs dictate. It fosters a far greater diversity of food experience for babies during the period of nutritional absorbency. (We'll talk more about what we call the period of nutritional absorbency later in "Starting Solid Foods: Taking Cues from Baby.")

Let's have a look at nutritional individuality from another view, that of the brain response. Food placed in the mouth evokes a brain response that is instantaneous, either for good or ill. This means that your brain immediately signals your digestive system, if food passes this brain response, to go-ahead and process and assimilate the food. However, if the food evokes a negative response from the bio-mind, the signal goes forth immediately to neutralize and eliminate the substance as completely and as quickly as possible. This brain response is quite subtle. Add to this that many adults and older children eat for many other and convoluted reasons than for uplifting or optimally healthful nutrition, and it is easy to see how this initial response to incompatible food is missed or ignored.

There seems to be a direct linkage between this innate brain response and children's abilities to intuitively select appropriate food. For others of us caught up in various problems of wrong eating, a more direct route of intuitive eating is still available to us—perhaps via reconnecting with our innate brain response to foods. Babies on living-foods diets tend to be connected to the immediate knowledge of what will work, i.e., in kinesiological terms, evoke the positive brain response in accord with their individual nutritional needs of the present moment, season, period of growth, and so forth.

To summarize, an enormous potential for difference in nutritional needs exists from person to person along with differences in the ability to digest and assimilate the needed foods. However, various foods have enormous differences in their inherent digestibility. Some things called "food" happen to be largely indigestible and toxic to various degrees, no matter what the individual needs or digestive powers might be. The human body's ability to compensate for toxic accumulations and other disturbances, in effect masking them, is another prime reason why it is so easy to ignore what are, for most people, usually only very subtle signs of toxic interference and metabolic blockage. We'll talk about the energetic compensatory system later on. Nutritional individuality needs to be discovered through our own experimentation. This will foster an awareness of which foods are more compatible for us. Organically grown, raw foods are inherently less toxic, less allergenic, more assimilable, and more supportive of a balanced, nutritional ecology. Raw foods consistently evoke the positive brain response for harmonious digestion and assimilation. Raw foods support order of both the visible and the larger mostly invisible levels of health and nutritional processes. Raw foods have the highest probability of being "right" for the widest range of nutritional needs. A simple, powerful tool becomes identifiable: The more raw-foods-dominant the diet becomes, the more stable this multidimensional thing called health and well-being remains.

The Non-toxic Child

Contemporary, naturopathic medicine recognizes toxic accumulation or interference in organs and tissues as a major causal factor in ill health. Exogenous toxins, or toxins that originate outside the body, are not entirely under our control. Importantly, we can drink filtered water, and eat locally grown, organic foods. We can move away from overly polluted, urban environments, and there is much else we can do; however, we will still be subjected to some degree of exogenous toxins.

Endogenous toxins originate inside the body as byproducts of metabolic processes such as digestion and regeneration. Levels of these toxins are much more subject to our control because the origin of much endogenous toxicity is dietary. Preservatives, flavor enhancers, colorings, growth hormones, pesticides, and antibiotic residues can all be retained in the organs, joints, and tissues. Biochemic and genetic individuality and pre-existing terrain imbalances determine how and where toxic accumulation will eventually affect us. One thing is clear: Toxic influences in the body eventually equal disturbance to health, bit by bit, little by little.

Organically grown foods in an uncooked state offer children a chance to remain toxin-free from the start of life. This is truly one priceless reward of starting your child with living foods. So many childhood problems are simply never encountered as a result of helping your child maintain this non-toxic state via the organic, raw-foods-dominant diet.

The Energetic Compensatory System and pH Balance

The human body is the ultimate detox machine. However, when this ability to eliminate toxins is overwhelmed, the body also has a tremendous capacity for storing toxins in the tissues. The body also has the innate ability to compensate for any ill effects or symptoms that might arise as a result of these toxic accumulations or other imbalances. In other words, the body is always attempting to minimize any interference, imbalance, or developing disease process by supplying more energy to the affected area, thus in effect compensating for the disturbance. This is all right and is one aspect of how balance is maintained. However, energy drain and a potentially deceptive masking of underlying problems can also result.

Another form of compensation and masking of underlying problems has to do with pH balance. In order to maintain the alkaline pH of the blood necessary for optimum health, the body will draw the alkalinizing minerals, such as calcium, from other areas, like bones, to provide the proper pH balance.

The body's reserves of calcium can be large in childhood, but if underlying conditions, in this case diet-induced acidifying conditions, are not corrected, the reserves naturally become depleted, various problems evolve, and on the surface all appears well. Standard testing, in this case for calcium deficiency, often only measures blood levels of calcium, which appear to be fine. Meanwhile, however, the underlying depletion of calcium from deeper levels of the body goes on unchecked. The mechanism of energetic compensation, a normal function when acute needs arise but a problematic mask over more serious chronic problems, embedded toxins, and creeping deficiencies, can give us an idea of how it is possible for underlying problems to go largely unnoticed until, suddenly, the body can no longer compensate. The mask fails, and symptoms of illness suddenly appear.

Breastfeeding as a Nutritional Model

Infants, babies, and young children often take twenty minutes to consume only several ounces of breast milk. During suckling the amount of milk in each "mouthful" is very small and has plenty of time to become thoroughly insalivated before being swallowed and further digested. The process of breastfeeding naturally dispenses small quantities and through suckling incorporates a very thorough mixing of milk and saliva.

Babies naturally continue a very thorough chewing of their first solid (pureed) foods. A small spoonful lasts a long time, if we let it. The first months of "solid" food are the perfect time to go with and promote this flow. Portions of one or two tablespoons are a good place to start. Give plenty of time between small spoonfuls. Observe how your child knows when she has had enough—the body language is unmistakable. When we eat too fast we miss, or learn to ignore, the signal of "enough" from the bio-mind. These are important habits, and the period of nutritional absorbency is the right time to begin their cultivation.

Other cultures and systems of nutritional thought have known this process. Macrobiotic practitioners, for instance, have always known pure food to be therapeutic in moderate to small quantities if chewed well and ultimately harmful if the quantity is too much, or if chewing is incomplete. The raw-foods-dominant school of thought also holds that less is more and that quality food thoroughly chewed and taken in strictly limited quantity works with oxygen, sunlight, and pure water to maintain balance and growth of the whole being that is just not possible when qualities and quantities consumed are not within certain limits.

Protein and Vitamin B-12

The B-12 issue is one that is critical to a successful and healthy vegan and raw-foods way of life.

— Gabriel Cousens, M.D.

Typically, most mainstream sources of nutritional information have stressed that vegans are prone to deficiency in both protein and vitamin B-12. In the case of protein this misinformation was based on studies done in the nineteen-twenties on the protein requirements of rats and wrongly assumed that human requirements were the same—the studies' legacy continues!

In the 1950s more advanced studies were done that determined the actual protein requirements of humans. Almost every unrefined vegetable food was found to have not only all eight essential amino acids but also the complete group of all the amino acids. This means that each vegetable protein is complete in its own right. Protein combining is therefore also not necessary. Protein from sprouts, nuts, greens, or tofu are each complete individually and will be used by the body as needed.

Quantity of protein is another issue with its own misinformational legacy. How much is enough? One way to approach this is to ask who, among all humans, requires the most protein? The obvious answer: babies. Babies are the most rapidly growing of human beings and thus have the greatest need for protein. Since the ideal baby food is mother's milk, its protein content provides a clue to how much is enough. One to two percent protein content is the norm for human breast milk. This is a surprise to a lot of folks. From this a more realistic idea of protein needs can be assessed. Protein excess, and the resultant toxic accumulations that can trigger metabolic problems, is common on the standard American diet. Even taking into account the differing protein needs of the various metabolic tendencies, far less protein is needed than tradition has preached, and vegetable sources definitely provide this lesser quantity in the right quality at the same time.

Vitamin B-12 is needed in very minute quantities and is stored for future use in the liver and muscles. Three to five millionths of a gram or micrograms are used daily. Vitamin B-12 in the vegan diet is controversial, and more research is needed. However, recent studies on vegan adults and children, using a more accurate standard of measurement, offer compelling indications that MOST vegans are far more at risk for serious B-12 deficiency than was previously thought.

Dr. Gabriel Cousens, M.D., one of the foremost researchers in the vegan and raw-foods movement has come to some important conclusions after reevaluating the B-12 issue. He has found that although B-12 is fairly plentiful in some vegan foods, like sea vegetables and spirulina, significant amounts of it are not useful to humans. Along with the human-active B-12 in these foods there is also a comparable amount of analog, or non-useful B-12. This analog B-12 competes for receptor sites in the body and can thus, in the long run, lead to deficiency.

Preliminary testing with the new standard for measuring B-12 levels seems to make a very urgent case for supplementation, especially for vegans and women who are pregnant. The following quote is from Dr. Cousen's recently released book *Spiritual Nutrition:* "The research conclusion is that it is a reasonably safe bet that about 80% of the vegan and live-food population, over time, runs the risk of B-12 deficiency...An even higher percentage of newborns run this risk."

It is important to note that newborns normally have only about 25 mcg. of B-12 in storage, compared to 2,000–3,000 mcg. stored in adults. Dr. Cousens recommends that during the time of breastfeeding

". . . perhaps all breastfeeding mothers should consider B-12 supplements for themselves and their infants."

One of the most important emphases of nutritional therapy is to correct intestinal dysfunction (dysbiosis), be it bacterial overgrowth, leaky gut syndrome, or lack of intestinal microvilli. These conditions, even if small in degree or masked by the energetic compensatory system, can severely limit absorption of all nutrients, especially vitamin B-12, whether one is vegan or not. Pharmaceutical drugs in general and general anesthetics in particular can dramatically increase the need for B-12 supplementation.

Given the new information that studies are confirming and the myriad stresses and health conditions in modern life that deplete this specific nutrient, Dr. Cousens' recommendations for all who are vegan, raw "foodists," also ring loudly for all parents and children. "It is well advised to supplement with an actual B-12 human-active supplement. There are vegan B-12 supplements which allow us to be totally successful, vegan, live fooders."

Origins of Synthetic Vitamins
and Nutritional Alchemy

Vitamins were first synthesized in the 1930s. Discovery of how to synthesize vitamins was a by-product of pharmaceutical research that was trying to better understand the pathways that vitamins take in the body in order to improve absorption of drugs. Many vitamins labeled as natural are still, at their core, synthetic products with small amounts of natural elements added in some cases. Food-based and food-grown vitamins are definitely more useable; however, the large majority of manufactured vitamins are, chemically speaking, a sort of mirror or inverse image of the real thing. Synthetics are thus able to fool the body, though for only a brief time; then they are quickly eliminated via the kidneys.

These vitamins can have their own beneficial effects if given for short periods and then discontinued once the desired effect has been achieved. They should be understood for what they really are—a separate category of foreign substances with their own potential drug effects and side effects. Synthetic thiamine and riboflavin have long been used to enrich refined flour, pasta, and cereal products. Studies have alleged that a gradual loss of fertility among western populations is the result of this kind of vitamin B-1 and B-2 supplementation. Pathological calcification in arteries and joints is believed by many researchers to be caused, in part, by the synthetic vitamin D that is widely used to fortify dairy products, and nowadays, even most non-dairy beverages.

Organically grown, raw, living foods have properties in their whole state that, as we know, dissipate or are destroyed by processing. When "vitamins" are seen for what they are, their use can also be limited—to achieving an effect in the near term when needed, not taken as a regular part of the daily diet. If you take a high-quality, food-grown type of vitamin supplement on a regular basis, it can be a good idea to take a break from it for a few weeks every once and a while.

Many vitamins are produced internally, by processes now generally known as nutritional alchemy. The goal of nutritional practice, and especially nutritional therapy, is to strengthen this innate process. Supplementation can allow the body to grow lazy in terms of its abilities to synthesize needed nutrients. Less is most often more where nutrition is concerned. A hundred units of vitamin A from raw vegetable juice are far more useful, without any side effects, than ten-thousand units of the mostly unusable, synthetic counterpart in pill form. We recommend elimination of all vitamin-enriched foods from the diet. Be very careful about vitamins where children are concerned.

Transitioning to Raw Foods: Detoxification and Regeneration

We understand that every life process is reversible. It might take from a few months to many years to make the transition back to the most fitting diet for the human being, but once we embark on the path, the benefits will be worth the effort.

— David Wolfe

In his book *The Sunfood Diet Success System,* author David Wolfe simply suggests eating basically whatever kind of organically grown, locally produced, raw, plant foods you like in whatever quantities you like as the best way to begin a living-foods diet. He also notes that finding a balance among leafy greens, sweet fruits, and fats is essential.

This total raw-foods diet is inherently non-toxic. However, once on this diet of all raw foods, extra pounds and stored toxins will begin to release into the system. This initial detoxification phase of the transition from a standard American diet to raw foods can take from several months to a year or two. Detoxification reactions can be severe and are to be avoided whenever possible. A slow steady detoxification is ideal. If difficulty arises, the process can be dramatically improved by use of complex homeopathic formulas designed specifically for the various phases of detoxification.

Increasing pure water intake is most helpful. Increasing the content of leafy greens in your diet over time, as well as homeopathic support for the major organs of elimination will strengthen the digestive system and ease the detoxification process, helping to smooth potentially uncomfortable reactions.

When detoxification is accomplished, regeneration will be naturally freer to occur as the natural next phase of the transition from a cooked to raw-foods diet. However, this process too can be difficult to start and maintain for some people. Again, homeopathic regeneration formulas are an indispensable aid, following significant detoxification, in establishing the regeneration process. Complex formulae are organ-specific and are designed to stimulate the pituitary gland to send its regeneration signals to the rest of the body.*

When children have been on a standard diet of processed foods for a number of years, they too can exhibit some signs of discomfort due to elimination of toxins from their bodies once on a raw-foods-dominant diet. Increasing pure water intake over an extended period will usually be enough to catch them up to a relatively non-toxic state. If you sense that toxins or imbalances are persisting, many forms of bioenergetic testing exist that can quickly and accurately pinpoint problem toxins and deficiencies that have become deeply seated and, for whatever reasons, do not seem to respond to diet and the cleansing effects of increased water intake over time.

---

*See "Practitioners and Testing," page 166, for more information on Future-plex Homeoenergetics.

Sea Vegetables
and the Homeopathic Ocean

*Everything that exists anywhere in the earth, or above it, finds
its way at last into the sea. Every element necessary for life is
present everywhere in the sea.*

— D.C. Jarvis, M.D.

Samuel Hahnemann discovered homeopathic principles late in the
eighteenth century. He proved that very small doses (microdoses) of
substances have therapeutic effects. But Hahnemann went further;
his special method of preparing microdoses from various substances
is generally known as "potentization."

Mainstream science has not yet fully explained how homeopathy
works. The process of potentization somehow accomplishes the development of subtle energetic patterns, also known as biosynerforms, a
term coined by Dr. Roy Martina, that the body can use in many ways
to restore balance. Homeopathy literally means similar disease. Hahnemann found that microdoses of herbs would produce a particular
pattern of symptoms when given to healthy people. Each herb, when
prepared homeopathically, produces its own characteristic pattern
of symptoms. When an ill person's symptom picture can be matched
with that produced by a homeopathic remedy, a curative process is
often begun. This principle is known as "like cures like." Hahnemann's
peculiar discovery, potentization, is a serial dilution and succussion
(percussive shaking) of prescribed parts of plant tincture and water. It

might go something like this: One part of a substance to be prepared is placed together with nine parts of the carrier, often distilled water and succussed one-hundred times. This diluted, succussed mixture is known as a 1x potency. To create a 2x potency the process is repeated by removing one part of the 1x solution, combining it with another nine parts water, and repeating the succussion. At approximately 24x potency none of the original physical substance is left in the preparation. However, potency increases the more the serial dilution/succussion, or potentization, continues.

Complex forms of homeopathy have been developed that employ substances other than the traditional plants used in classical homeopathy. Minerals, for instance, that have undergone potentization have unique properties. Embryonic plant buds, at low potencies, have unique rejuvenative effects. Following the principle of like cures like, many toxic substances have also been processed homeopathically to produce toxin-specific remedies.

The world ocean has become a repository for all manner of substances, both beneficial and toxic. This ocean, and its million miles of coastline worldwide, is the natural laboratory in which dilution and succussion of this complex mix of elements is constantly taking place. Looking at the world ocean through this homeopathic lens, it is easy to understand how healing potential is present in the sea and sea vegetables via, among other things, the ongoing, natural homeopathic process.

Nori and dulse, especially nori sheets, are fave-rave snacks among the kiddies. Playing on the beach and breathing sun-charged ocean mist is also a favorite. Sea vegetables appear to be the "green foods" that work to continuously rebalance the human organism with the most oomph from many angles. On ocean-going ships in the past, sea water, for instance, was often used in place of blood for transfusions. Its mineral content and general composition is almost identical to human blood.

We recommend that you incorporate sea vegetables into your diet. Sea vegetables are superfoods in their own special right whose dynamic influence for vibrant health and probable proactive, homeopathically supplemented, panacea-like qualities deserve further exploration. You can rotate among the several varieties. Not only is vitamin B-12 present in many sea vegetables, but also existent are astounding arrays of elements, both nutritional and healing, as yet unidentified but predictable via the above mentioned natural homeopathic process. If you garden, incredibly healthful foods can be grown in soil where sea vegetables are either prepared biodynamically or through regular composting worked into the soil. Forewarned is forearmed: Enjoy the beach!

❦ RADIATION, CHILDREN, AND SEA VEGETABLES

Infants and young children are among the most susceptible groups when it comes to the various forms of radiation exposure; the other groups are the elderly and people in poor health. The so-called "safe doses" of radiation that have traditionally been issued by the government are meaningless because radiation is cumulative.

The raw-foods-dominant diet is a good place to start for protection against the dangers of radiation. First, it promotes a high level of health, generally reducing susceptibility to radiation. Second, raw foods keep the body more alkaline, which also reduces susceptibility. Third, a raw-foods-dominant diet has a far higher mineral profile, which is also key in protection against radiation.

Sea vegetables in particular have the ability to chelate or draw radioactive particles to them and pass them out of the body harmlessly. Sodium alginate is the chelator found most prolifically in the kelp family that removes the most radioactive material. The kelp family includes kelp, hijiki, arame, and wakame. Sea vegetables can also chelate plutonium, lead, cesium, and cadmium. Sea vegetables contain all minerals and trace elements that humans require and are high in chlorophyll, enzymes, vitamin A, and all the B vitamins. As mentioned earlier, they are a great source of B-12. The merchant, Maine Coast Sea Vegetables, is an excellent source of sun-dried sea vegetables. Maine Coast monitors their harvest extensively for the presence of toxins.

Putting It All Together:
Ideas and Guidance
for the Individual Health Plan

*Food must be a spiritual idea. It must be an idea of substance
and supply . . . there is an intelligence within us, which will guide
us into a proper diet. Since each is an individual, the intaking of
food is an individual idea and an individual approach to reality.
Whatever our individual system needs to make it harmonious,
Intelligence will guide us to.*

— Ernest Holmes, *The Science of Mind*

We can think of genuinely well-rounded health as occurring through
four overlapping domains: spinal alignment/structural, nutrition,
emotions/spirit, and circulatory or cardiovascular health. Our individual development of a raw-foods-dominant dietary lifestyle will, over
time, dramatically assist the progressive balance of the other three
domains (structure, emotions, and cardiovascular). However, beyond
the positive influence of living nutrition each of these three domains
has special practices that, when used together, synergistically assist in
an accelerated achievement of more balanced levels of health.

It is not within the scope of this book to catalog the healthcare
modalities available for work in the structural, spiritual, or cardiovascular domains—however, careful and conscious attention to these

aspects of health is essential to putting together an Individual Health Plan (IHP). Here are some suggestions to get you started in the working formulation of your IHP. Phone consultations and personal training are also available from the authors.

❧ STRUCTURAL INTEGRITY/REPROGRAMMING THE SPINE

Many styles and systems of bodywork attempt to improve structural integrity. Yoga, biokinesiology, and other self-help methods of position-release exercise are highly effective in the proactive maintenance of both skeletal and muscular/ligamentous integrity. For more primary care, however, Network Spinal Analysis™ offers what many feel is a highly effective and refined multidimensional approach to healthcare ostensibly through the structural domain. Network Spinal Analysis is often very affordable and is simply great for kids.

Both yogic exercise/breathing and network entrainment of the nervous system/breathing can easily overlap with the emotional and spiritual domain because they are conducive to states of mental quietude, meditation, and the retracing and release of old traumas that can underlie structural imbalance and thus affect the whole of wellbeing.

❧ PSYCHOSOMATICA

Emotional or psychosomatic influence is present to some degree in most if not all health disturbances. A calm and relatively quiet mind is ultimately as important to health as the yogic postures, spinal entrainments, aerobic exercise, and living foods that need to go with and support it. Unfortunately, development of emotional calm or even spiritual presence through quieting of the mind is somewhat of a lost art. After age one or two, children can easily begin learning it when they can see it being modeled by others.

✤ NUTRITION AGAIN

The nutritional domain has its special tools in addition to the foundational daily practice of a raw-foods-dominant diet. The overarching idea here is that we are moving from standard aberrant practices of nutrition and health to much more refined practices of the same. Initially, a transitional phase requires some degree of adjustment, often considerable in adults and older children, that involves detoxification; replenishment of depleted reserves on several levels; restoration of nervous and regenerative function; and the emotional acceptance, reorientation, and growth needed to integrate the transition. Bioenergetic testing, Terrain testing, Contact Reflex Analysis, Computerized Electro Dermal Screening (CEDS), and homeopathic supplementation are very economic, effective, and paint an accurate picture of nutritional and metabolic disturbances. Please see the "References, Further Reading, and Resources" section for how to find bioenergetic, nutritional, and terrain testing in your area.

The need for a plan, however informal, is essential during this important transition. This transitional period, and the rebuilding and balancing of the internal ecology that occurs with testing or not, is usually at least six months to a year and a half. It is a work of faith in progress and need not be rushed or agonized over. How long this transitional period takes depends basically on three things: the size and depth of the toxic load to be eliminated; the degree of disturbance among the organs, tissues, and internal terrain; and lastly, the degree of individual determination and vision to achieve wellness.

Doing for yourself and your loved ones what no one else can—maintaining internal calm, eating right, keeping the spine free of interference, and enjoying some form of physical exercise—is simultaneously a joy and a challenging need to be fulfilled in order to stay whole in today's world.

The Last Word: Water

*Chronic cellular dehydration painfully and prematurely kills.
Its initial outward manifestations have until now been labeled
as diseases of unknown origin.*

— F. Batmanghelidj, M.D.

In terms of health and wellness water really is the first and the last word. For many reasons, some very well known and some still very mysterious, it is absolutely critical to drink adequate water every day (a minimum of 4–5 eight-ounce glasses).

Much like living food being compromised by various forms of processing including overheating, water too can be rendered mostly useless, not easily absorbed by cells by processing including heating, chlorination, and so forth. There is then more to pure water than simply the absence of pollutants; the natural hexagonal structure of water needs to be present for water to most rapidly penetrate into the body's cells. Water ionizers help structure water and increase the alkalinity, which in turn increases available minerals and oxygen for the body. Keep in mind that raw fruits and vegetables are naturally high in structured water. These foods are a fine source of structured water intake. High content of structured water is yet another important benefit of the raw-foods-dominant diet.

Unstructured water that consists of conglomerates too large to easily get into cells must be re-structured in the body—this also takes a lot of energy and time. Structured alkaline water can penetrate cells much more quickly, thus improving metabolic function, nutrient delivery, waste removal, and of course the actual hydration of cells.

Remember that typical aging is definitely accompanied by a slow but steady decrease in the total water content of the body—estimated to be as much as 80% at birth and as little as 50% in old age. Infants and young children can become dehydrated more easily than adults. It seems that if the mother is drinking pure water everyday (4–5 eight-ounce glasses) then breastfeeding babies also get enough. After six months of age, 2–3 ounces of water several times a day is a good start. Formula-fed babies need more water to help eliminate the toxins found in cow's milk. As our kids grow and mature, we must always cultivate their awareness of the need for water.

The well-known facts—that the human body is 75% water and that water is needed for digestion, elimination of wastes, and regulation of the body temperature—are just the beginning where water is concerned. The roots of the many and multidimensional functions and actions of water in and around the body are very deep, very subtle. They have always been this way, and yet we hardly notice them. Distribution of available water in the body takes place through a very complex system. Similar to the way in which we have learned to ignore the brain response that subtly informs us which foods will currently work for the body, so too we have learned, in large part via the standard American diet, to ignore the basic signals for water. In many cases this disconnection is so extreme that thirst is often interpreted as a signal to eat!

Both reverse-osmosis and distilled water are widely available, very pure, and generally close to neutral in pH. Countertop water ionizers* that quickly and economically produce purified alkaline water are also becoming more widely available. In extensive Japanese research over the past two decades, alkaline water has proven incredibly effective

---

*See page 174 in the "References, Further Reading, and Resources" section for suppliers of water ionizers.

in reversing aging and over time healing all manner of chronic conditions. Alkaline water is critical to the ability to easily and consistently balance the many acidifying stresses of modern life and prevent mineral depletion. It also promotes oxygenation of the whole system and clear nerve function. Some practitioners recommend restructuring, or naturalizing of water that has been heated by distillation or destructured by electrolysis, by sitting it in natural light for a few hours, which is very mysterious.

The last word is to drink water regularly: morning, noon, and evening. Ionized alkaline water is one good way to go. Over time, the consumption of pure water will slowly but surely work toward a thorough cleansing and rejuvenation of the whole body. It is a key component in keeping your children toxin free. It is also key to the success of any individual health plan. Reconnect with your thirst and hold it near!

Part II

Foods, Recipes, and Activities

by Michaela Lynn

Keys to Balance:
Healthy Thoughts for Healthy Eating

Living foods are inherently supportive of life. But even if our diet is 100% raw, if our thoughts surrounding these foods do not affirm life, we end up missing out on the very quality of life we are seeking. Key to the experience of joyful balance is honoring all aspects of ourselves— our whole selves. As we set new dietary goals for ourselves, it is our highest good to be at peace with that within us that seeks to meet all of our inter-connected needs: physical, social, emotional, mental, and spiritual. Here are affirming thoughts for each of these:

Mental: Whatever is nourishing, healing, loving, and inspiring—think upon these things.

Physical: Rather than giving intellect full reign over what is best, expecting the body to solely obey its will, make a point to check in with your body. The body wills to live, to experience life's pleasures, to be blessed. Take time to be quiet enough to hear its subtle messages. Listen to its likes and dislikes, symptoms, and cravings. Before eliminating major dietary components or even food favorites from your family diet, replace them with others. (If you are vegan or desire to be, see our previous article on vitamin B-12.)

Spiritual: I grew up in a spiritual community where outings to fast-food restaurants were a ritual. We would sit down with our doughnuts, sodas, burgers, and fries, and someone would utter the prayer, "Bless this food to our bodies' use." I find these memories somewhat amusing now, but within them I also find wisdom: Whatever your present diet, bless it! When you think about it, all foods have something to offer us: energy, pleasure, and sustenance of life, to name a few. What about the foods that give the effects of sluggishness, hyper-activity, or depression, or contribute to obesity and other forms of disease? These too have value. They are our opportunities, if you will, to make changes, to seek a new relationship with how we nourish our bodies. Rather than categorize some foods as good and others as bad (you know, angel vs. devil's food cake, sinfully decadent, guilt-free meals, etc.), bless *all* of your food choices for the wisdom they offer you. This is a helpful first step in releasing the habits you wish to change. Spiritual beliefs that are guilt producing, shaming, judgmental, or self-righteous are less than life affirming. They alienate us from parts of ourselves, our family members, and others. If you find yourself hiding food or scolding or punishing yourself or your family over food choices, this is doubtfully the healthy lifestyle you are striving for. Counseling may be very helpful for getting to the root cause of this issue. Relax, love yourself, and bless all that you eat.

Social: We all have the need for loving connections with others. Our children need to socialize with other children. Share your favorite recipes, live in dietary tolerance, and check in with your social self (and that within your child) when making decisions about social events for your family. Our own family dietary practice is sometimes somewhat different at home than what we may eat in the homes of others.

Children's need for autonomy: Bless your children's decisions even when they differ from your own. Children are doing their job when they are curious, when they explore that which is other than what their parents choose for them. Our kids follow within them what drives them to be their own persons and to honor their whole selves: to assess the world around them for themselves and to live out their own destinies. When they step out on their own, they seek firsthand knowledge such as: What feels good in my body? Why does my friend like this? We are most helpful when we ask them what they think about their experiences and value what they say, before we tell them what we think. *Allow for experimentation with foods.* They need this! And if you do not permit it, they will sneak food, obsess over it, and experience guilt over their choices. Live a healthy example and trust in their instincts. Here are two encouraging stories:

1. When I was a kid, I saw a TV ad for a processed, snack-pudding pie. The pie looked incredible and the child eating it in pure bliss. I *had* to have one. Mama wasn't one for such blatant junk food, but I mustered up my courage one day at the grocery store to ask for one. She said yes! That alone felt great! I tore the plastic wrapping off as soon as I got out to the car. The pie looked noticeably different than the one in the ad—it didn't have that fresh, out-of-the-oven look. I tried it anyway, and I was thoroughly disappointed. It didn't taste at all like I had fantasized, and I never ate one again.

2. My mother avoided processed sugar, while my grandmothers stocked up on it. When I was at grandma's, I binged on all the goodies. I remember noticing on my own that my body felt yucky. Then I would get the urge to eat carrot sticks, which would help me feel better.

Experimentation with food need not be open-ended. When my two-and-a-half-year-old daughter asks me about foods that have resulted from animal suffering, for example, I honor her curiosity by saying, "I can see how that would look fun to you because of the picture on the wrapper, the colors, etc. I don't feel comfortable buying this one, but I want to find something else new and fun for you to try." Then we go and look for something animal-friendly that has similar appeal. As she gets older and probes further, she and I will have some heart-to-heart talks about how we can help our animal friends who are suffering.

Clean-plate club? Many of us were made to eat all of the food put on our plates. We sat there and stared at the liver and onions until they were either choked down or secretly fed to the dog. We're finding now, however, that such authoritarian feeding practices contribute to obesity and other eating disorders. What to do with a case of the "finickies"? Read the sections on "Toddler Foods" and "Recipes for Children" for some helpful tips.

Many children do not want to eat any meat. Some babies refuse it from the start, while older children may respond in compassion or disgust once they have learned where the food has come from. "Teens are old enough to recognize animal suffering and young enough to want to do something about it," says Carol Adams, author of *Help! My Child Stopped Eating Meat!* Don't worry, there is no need to pressure your child to eat meat and every reason to support him/her in finding healthful alternatives. If you are concerned over meeting your child's nutritional needs and feel unequipped, consult a nutritionist with vegetarian expertise. Living foods will feed your young vegetarian well! Soaked nuts and seeds are excellent sources of protein, for example, while fresh greens, dried fruits, and spirulina are all high in iron. (Read the "Superfoods and Babies" and "Recipes for Children" sections for more ideas and info.)

Basic Tools and Equipment

❧ EQUIPMENT

We recommend starting out with the following three machines in your raw foods kitchen:

- Blender

- Juicer

- Dehydrator

- Electric coffee grinder/food processor

Blender: The blender is instrumental in preparing baby foods and making soups, sauces, smoothies, and dips. The Vita-Mix is probably the most well-known, high-power blender on the market. If you've had to replace your blender numerous times, one of these hearty appliances might be a great investment. All of our recipes that call for blender use, however, can be prepared using a standard blender; a glass container is preferred.

Juicer: Several high-quality juicers are on the market, such as the Champion and the Green Power machine. The Green Power machine, for example, juices wheat grass and any other greens. (It also can make pasta, bread dough, sorbets, and sauces.) However, for economical fruit and vegetable juicing, you can't beat the Juice Man Juicer, which typically sells for about $70.00 (a fraction of the cost of the more heavy-duty juicers.) It could be a good way to get started. You may prefer, however, to invest in the better-quality juicers, which have a long warrantee and tend to extract more of the juice from fruits and vegetables. (In the long run, this may save expenses on buying produce and/or replacing your juicer.)

Dehydrator: The Excalibur dehydrator, which comes in four-tray or larger size, is useful for making raw cookies, crackers, and fruit leather, and for gently warming foods without the loss of enzymes. With a dehydrator, you can also dry your own fresh fruits and vegetables for storage. Foods can be set under the sun to dry or sometimes placed in a warm, conventional oven set on the lowest heat. The sun method and the Excalibur are the most reliable for ensuring that temperatures remain below 115°F.

Electric coffee grinder/food processor: In addition to these three machines, you may also want to have an electric coffee grinder for finely grinding small amounts of dried herbs and seeds. It can be especially useful for grinding flax seeds fresh. A food processor is also handy for grating, slicing, or chopping large amounts of foods as well as making pates, dips, and desserts.

⚘ Tools

Graters: The common box grater is indispensable. It is used for standard grating as well as very fine grating, which can effectively puree small amounts of fresh fruits into sauces fit for babies.

Wide-mouth glass jars: We use these for sprouting, soaking, and pickling. Plastic screen tops can also be purchased for draining sprouts, or you can simply use a square of mesh screening with a rubber band to hold it in place atop the jar. Higher-tech sprouting systems are also available for purchase (see "References, Further Reading, and Resources" section).

Saladecco Spiralizer: This tool is not essential but adds fun to food preparation, giving raw veggies a boost in kid-appeal. It slices squash, zucchini, cucumbers, and beets into angel hair pasta-thin strands. Once an adult has put it together, a child can help by turning the crank. We don't have it listed in our kid's tool section, however, because the blades are very sharp when unassembled.

Miscellaneous tools: Other raw-kitchen desirables may include: a good set of sharp knives; measuring cups and spoons; cutting boards; glass pie plates; and several wooden, stainless steel, or glass mixing bowls.

✴ KITCHEN TOOLS FOR KIDS

One of the best ways to foster a lifetime love for living foods in our children is by including them as much as we can in the growing and preparing of their own meals and snacks. The children not only gain awareness, self-confidence, and skills that will follow them into adulthood, but they are also able to do what they love best—spend time with you!

One of the great advantages to not cooking food is that the hazards of hot ovens or boiling pots are eliminated, helping to create a more child-friendly space for little helpers. Eating raw can be as pure and simple as picking and eating straight from the vine, but it oftentimes involves preparations such as chopping, juicing, and blending. Sharp knives and electrical appliances can also tend to leave children out of mealtime preparations. Here's a list of kid-friendly tool ideas for you and your budding young raw-foods chef:

1. *Child-sized safety scissors:* These round-tip snips will cut nori sheets as they do paper and are perfect for shearing wheat grass from a flat or garden patch.

2. *Manual wheat grass juicer:* Costing somewhere around $90.00, this is the priciest tool on the list. I initially bought mine to reduce

my dependency on electrical appliances, later finding it to be a fun tool for juicing with little ones. Children are intrigued by the mechanics of turning the hand crank and watching the dark green juice run out through the spout. It doesn't do much more for fruits and veggies than make them into mush, but it does work quite well with wheat grass and other herbs such as fresh parsley or mint.

3. *Manual citrus juicer:* Glass juicers with a child-sized handle are listed in the Montessori catalog (see "References, Further Reading, and Resources" section), but plastic or stainless steal might be more preferable as they're more likely to withstand a drop to the floor. The knob-handled, hard-wood variety work great too. If your family uses lots of limes, you may also want a manual juicer specifically designed for mini-limes. They are common in Mexico and look like a cross between a citrus juicer and garlic press.

4. *Wire "egg" slicer:* Do you have one of these? They're not just for hard-boiled eggs! This little gadget slices mushrooms, strawberries, kiwis (peeled), and bananas (peeled) without nicking little fingers. (The wires are not strong enough for harder fruits and veggies, however, and will break if these foods are attempted.)

5. *Melon baller:* Helping with their finer motor skills, kids can sculpt their favorite melon into little ball-shaped bites.

6. *Garlic press:* This familiar no-knife tool is user friendly for kids and saves you the time of mincing cloves of garlic.

7. *Cookie cutters:* For special fun cut raw fruits and veggies like cucumbers, apples, or jicama into playful shapes.

8. *Mortar and pestle:* Ceramic or stone ones seem to work best. The mortar and pestle can take the place of an electric coffee grinder, crushing dried herbs and seeds.

9. *Manual coffee grinder:* Hardwood and metal, it has an adjustable grinding mechanism. They are listed in the Montessori catalog.

10. *Veggie peeler:* This is to be used under adult supervision for the younger child, as it is not completely nick-proof. I use mine mostly for making carrot curls for topping salads.

11. *Safety grater:* Also listed in the Montessori catalog, this manual grater has a safety feature for kids. The grating attachment fits atop a measuring cup, which catches the veggie shreds and acts as a protective cover for their little fingers.

12. *Measuring cups and spoons:* A part of most every modern kitchen, a set of each is a helpful tool for learning about fractions and measurements.

13. *Sprouting jars and screens:* Also listed in the basic tools, using these simple sprouting tools is a perfect way for children to observe the life of food.

14. *Push-down apple slicer:* By holding onto the handled sides of this simple slicer, it can be positioned over an apple's top and pushed down through the bottom, separating the wedges from the core. An adult needs to assist the younger child to ensure that their fingers stay wrapped around the handles of the tool.

Kitchen Hygiene: Keeping It Natural

For many of us, cooking with extreme temperatures is the most familiar method of "sanitizing" food. Concerns over food safety can then naturally arise as we begin preparing meals without the application of heat. This can be of particular concern when preparing foods for infants (who've not yet built up their own antibodies) or when traveling to another country where there may be parasites and/or bacteria that are foreign to our own immunities. Observing a raw-foods diet, however, can actually improve our standard of food-safety.

One reason it can is that the living-foods diet does not traditionally include flesh-foods, dairy, or eggs, products which are found most productive of food poisoning. Meat, for example, is likely to have been tainted by fecal-borne bacteria either on the farm or in the slaughterhouse. And according to the U.S. Center for Disease Control and Prevention (CDC) 70–90% of all chickens are carriers of campylobacter jejuni, the pathogen that is the most common bacterial cause of diarrheal illness in the U.S. The CDC has also estimated that one out of every fifty consumers will be exposed to a salmonella-contaminated egg each year.

Pregnant women are often advised by their physicians and midwives to avoid eating deli foods, hot dogs, and cold cuts as well as soft cheeses (such as feta, brie, Camembert, bleu, and Mexican style cheeses). These and other meat, dairy, and processed foods often harbor the bacteria listeria, which survives refrigerator temperatures and sometimes even deep-freezes. Pregnant women in particular are at higher risk of getting the infection listeriosis, which can also be passed to her unborn child.

The living-foods diet also supports breastfeeding, which is naturally more sanitary than using bottles and artificial nipples, which often carry bacteria even after washing.

Observing a raw-foods diet not only minimizes our exposure to these contaminants, but it also builds our bodies' resistance to infection. With heightened nutrition and less of our bodies' energy spent on simple digestion, the stronger our immune system becomes (along with our ability to detoxify). As our level of vitality rises, we also become a less-hospitable host to parasites. If our digestion is optimal, parasites will not proliferate but will be terminated by concentrated digestive secretions.

Living foods, by their very nature, are indeed more perishable than processed foods that can sit on the shelf for months. Here are some basic raw-food safety guidelines:

1. Wash hands thoroughly with soap and water before preparing food (and after each time you are interrupted to change a diaper, wipe a nose, cover a cough, handle money, etc.).

2. Wash foods thoroughly before preparation. Soak leafy greens to remove accumulated soil and then rinse at least three times. (This is most important with store-bought produce as it may contain mold and other toxins. That which is picked from your home garden has a much higher standard of purity and freshness.)

3. Remove all rotting or blemished spots on produce. If fruits and veggies are organic and well cleaned there is no need to peel them, sacrificing added nutrients and fiber.

4. The living-foods diet is traditionally vegetarian. If animal products are currently a part of your diet, use extra care not to allow your raw fruits and vegetables to be cross contaminated. Make sure that all meats are cooked thoroughly. This helps prevent contracting

parasites. Everything that touches raw meat, dairy, or eggs, during food preparation needs to be washed thoroughly in hot, soapy water, insuring that utensils that have touched raw animal products do not come into contact with foods that will not be cooked. Use different cutting boards for raw fish and other meat than you do for fruits and veggies. Wash hands again after handling raw animal products. Wipe down your work surface area as well as cleaning the sink.

5. Fresh juices are best consumed soon after they are extracted, rather than storing them until the next day in the refrigerator. Commercial unpasteurized juices (bottled, as opposed to juices that are made fresh at home or on site at a juice bar) are not considered to be safe for young children.

6. Raw honey is not recommended for babies under the age of one year because of cases of infant botulism that have been linked to its use.

7. Fermented foods such as sauerkraut, nut/seed cheeses, kefirs, and yogurts are popular raw foods because of their distinctive flavors and digestive-aiding cultures. They are not recommended for babies under the age of one year, however, because they can also carry unfriendly bacteria.

✺ Recipes for Natural Cleaning

By using non-toxic products, children can be invited to clean right along side of you. Cleaning up doesn't always have to be a chore. Spray bottles, sponges, and bubbles are all good candidates for a younger child's play. Play some fun music like "I've got to be clean" by Guster (on the album *For the Kids* by various artists) and go ahead and get silly and sudsy.

Fruit and Veggie Soak Solutions

1. 1 tablespoon apple-cider vinegar per 1 gallon of water or ¼ cup apple-cider vinegar per sinkful. For ridding any parasites that could be present on your produce, soak raw fruits and vegetables in this solution for 15 minutes.

2. 1 tablespoon 3% Hydrogen Peroxide (H_2O_2) per 1 gallon water, or ¼ cup H_2O_2 per sinkful. Soak raw fruits and veggies in this solution for 15 minutes. *Alternative method:* Spray 3% H_2O_2 directly on produce, wait 1–2 minutes, then rinse. This will remove parasites as well as pesticide residue.

3. 2 tablespoons salt and juice of ½ lemon per sinkful of water will also act as a pesticide wash for non-organic produce.

Vinegar as a Disinfectant

Studies have shown that a straight 5% solution of vinegar kills 99% of bacteria, 82% of mold, and 80% of viruses. White distilled vinegar is preferred, as apple-cider vinegar can leave stains. Spray bottles can be filled with straight 5% vinegar to clean and deodorize countertops, cutting boards, and sinks. The vinegar smell will go away within a few hours.

Herbal Anti-Bacterial Hand Soap

Lavender oil and tea tree oil both have natural anti-bacterial properties. If anti-bacterial soap is desired add 5–10 drops of either oil to your regular hand soap. Many natural soaps already contain these oils. Dr. Bronner's Castile soap, for example, comes in both varieties.

All-Purpose Spray Cleaner

½ teaspoon washing soda
Squirt of liquid soap
2 cups of hot tap water

Combine ingredients in spray bottle and shake until washing soda is dissolved. Apply and wipe with a rag or sponge.

Tea Tree Oil Spray

2 teaspoons tea tree oil
2 cups water

Combine in spray bottle and shake. Spray on moldy or mildewed areas. Do not rinse. This spray has a long shelf life.

Living Foods and Pregnancy:
A Lot to Be Said for Women's Intuition

Now with every new moon
Safe inside your cocoon
A strand more of your body is spun
As does mine own grow
Ample, round, and aglow
As fruit ripening under the sun.
Tis as sweet, blessed one,
My love for you.

> — Michaela Lynn, from the poem "Angel's Secrets"
>   written to daughter Quinn in utero

One of the first ways that babies learn about flavors is through
amniotic fluid and breast milk. We're finding that foods eaten
during pregnancy and lactation can influence a baby's willing-
ness to accept those foods later.

> — Julie Mennella, taste researcher at Monell Chemical Senses
>   Center in Philadephia, *Parents* magazine, March 2004

As we seek to know better our bodies and to honor them with living foods, pregnancy endows us with profound opportunities. A time of new beginnings, we often have a fresh outlook on our lives and added motivation to make healthy changes to our lifestyles. When we are pregnant, our bodies tend to get our attention. Perplexing food aversions are followed by ravenous cravings, we often feel more fatigue, and our emotions sweep over us with strengthened momentum. During pregnancy, we are given a peak of opportunity to tune into our body's needs. These include the specific needs of the fetus who now shares her mother's body.

Research suggests that "morning sickness" for example, could very well be our bodies' way of guiding us in the avoidance of eating various foods. In her book *Protecting Your Baby-to-Be*, Margie Profet presents a strong case that the symptom of nausea common in early months of pregnancy (when the risk of miscarriage is highest) serves to guard the embryo from potentially harmful levels of plant toxins. These include vegetables such as onions, garlic, broccoli, mushrooms, cabbage, and potatoes, as well as spices, and most herbs, tea, coffee, cola, and barbecued and fried foods.

This theory may offer some insight for women who experience difficulty eating their typical raw fare during pregnancy. I remember my own first trimester, walking into the Tree of Life Café, surrounded by herbaceous gourmet dishes. All of these great nutritious foods to choose from, but the only offering I could bring myself to nibble on were a few carrot and celery sticks. The peppery greens, fresh herbs and spices, and even the cold-pressed oils that I favored before pregnancy now suddenly made my stomach churn. For those first few weeks, the only food I seemed to be able to eat of any real quantity was fruit. Interestingly enough, fresh, raw fruit is the food that Profet concludes is best suited for the first three months of pregnancy.

It is after the initiation of first-trimester nausea that our desire for food generally begins to diversify. We may even find ourselves with some surprising cravings. As with morning sickness, these new food urges can also help to guide us in dietary decisions. Maybe you've heard Great Depression stories of pregnant women having the urge to eat dirt. This and cravings for other strange items (also referred to as "pica") have long been associated with the lack of essential minerals. More commonly, our hunger leads us to food sources. Sometimes we reach for whole and natural foods, but what about the strong urges for the "junk" or nutrient-depleted foods? In *Juicing for Life: A Guide to the Health Benefits of Fresh Fruit and Vegetable Juicing*, authors Cherie Calbom and Maureen Keane offer some advice (recommendations are general, not exclusive to pregnant women): Finding the root cause of these strange food urges means "recognizing that even though you are ravenously hungry for a whole quart of pistachio ice cream or both bags of pretzels, that isn't what your body needs biochemically. The chances are strong that it needs something very different."

Calbom and Keane explain five common types of food cravings and the possible real nutritional need behind them: Cravings for chocolates and other sweets, for starters (a fine place to start!), often indicate deficiency in the mineral chromium found in foods such as apples, green pepper, whole wheat, carrots, spinach, and brewer's yeast. Craving sweets may also be a sign of the need for additional protein. It makes sense that these cravings might suddenly appear (or intensify) during pregnancy—a time when our biological requirement for protein is higher. In *Conscious Eating*, Gabriel Cousens, M.D., says that an expectant mothers' protein intake needs to increase by at least 30 grams, to approximately 60–75 grams per day depending on one's constitutional type. Abundant sources of vegetable protein are: sprouted nuts and seeds, and whole grains and legumes (beans, split peas, or lentils). In the book *Sunfood Success Diet*, David Wolfe recommends eating date-covered almonds (remove the pits and replace with raw almonds) when chocolate bar cravings strike. These sweet protein nuggets are very satisfying. Craving chocolate may also be a craving for magnesium. For this reason, raw, peruvian olives may be helpful.

Salty food cravings on the other hand are often caused by adrenal stress, which may result from caffeine use or other factors. Calbom and Keane advise reducing table salt and increasing organic potassium, such as in parsley, garlic, spinach, and carrots. Other nutrients that support the adrenal glands are pantothenic acid (found in broccoli, cauliflower, and kale), vitamin C (kale and other leafy greens, parsley, bell pepper, and citrus), vitamin B-6 (kale, spinach, turnip greens, and sweet pepper), magnesium (beet greens, spinach, parsley, and garlic) and zinc (gingerroot, parsley, potato, garlic, and carrot). Regular table salt is easily replaced by sea salt or Celtic salt, which are more natural forms of salt. Bragg's Liquid Amino Acids is another healthful alternative. It may be important to note that cravings for salt can also be a sign of high blood pressure, diabetes, or other serious health problems.

If you are experiencing ice cravings (also called pagophagia), it's a good idea to have your blood tested for anemia. Anemia often results from deficiency in iron, vitamin B-12, and/or folic acid, which our bodies need more of during pregnancy. Plant foods high in iron include: pumpkin seeds, sunflower seeds, millet and other whole grains, parsley, almonds, leafy greens, legumes, sorghum molasses, and dried fruits. Foods that are high in vitamin C (see list above) are also key to increasing the body's absorption of iron. In *Pregnancy, Children and the Vegan Diet*, Michael Klaper, M.D., tells us that, "sixty milligrams of vitamin C increases the absorption of the iron in corn by five times!. . . Green leafy vegetables (which contain both iron and vitamin C)," he says, "are especially valuable foods during pregnancy." Other vitamin C-rich foods: "turnip greens, tomatoes, and cabbage," say Klaper, "are especially good to combine with iron-rich foods." Because the iron-absorption rate is different for each person, Klaper does not recommend uniform supplementation for every woman. "Excess iron tablets can cause stomach irritation and can actually be toxic to mother and fetus."

When I was diagnosed with mild anemia during my own pregnancy, I was able to correct the imbalance through regular fruit and vegetable juicing (iron- and C-rich), as well as taking the liquid herbal supplement Floradex (available in health-food stores). The reduction or elimination of milk products can also be helpful, as dairy has been shown to inhibit the absorption of iron. Foods rich in folic acid include: black-eyed peas, rice, wheat germ, legumes, asparagus, walnuts, dark leafy greens, and dates. "Ample helpings of broccoli, kale, collards, or spinach, as well as one or two dried dates every few days will insure the recommended one milligram daily intake throughout pregnancy," says Klaper. (More information on vitamin B-12 is given in Part I.)

Peanut butter cravings may mean that your body hungers for foods rich in copper. This includes peanuts, but because they are roasted before being ground into butter, the chances of rancid oils are high. This is why eating peanut butter can result in indigestion. Peanuts are also often avoided because they commonly contain of aflatoxins (a carcinogenic mold). If you're craving peanut butter by the spoonful right out of the jar, here are some ways to diversify: brazil nuts, hazelnuts, walnuts, pecans, split peas, buckwheat, gingerroot, coconut, apple, carrot, and garlic are all foods high in copper. Peanut butter cravings could also mean that your body is simply asking for healthy fats (for more info on these fats see the "Toddler Foods" section). A high-salt diet can also bring on cravings for fatty foods. Also try raw, salted, pumpkinseed butter (available through Nature's First Law; see the "References, Further Reading, and Resources" section). It tastes very similar to natural peanut butter.

Last on the Calbom/Keane common-craving list is the urge for something sour. "Your body may need acetic acid to help detoxify a chemical produced from decaying proteins," says the author-team. This chemical builds up in the body due to putrefying foods in the intestinal tract. Calbom and Keane advise clearing up any issues of constipation or if that's not the problem, drinking one teaspoon of fresh lemon juice in water (to provide the acetic acid). They also recommend chlorophyll-rich green juices as well as foods high in riboflavin (vitamin B-2). B-2 rich foods, such as almonds, mushrooms, wheat germ, wild rice, millet, wheat bran, and brewer's yeast, aid the metabolism of acetic acid.

In addition to hinting at our nutritional needs, food cravings can have other implications as well. Many people with food allergies, for example, report that the foods to which they are sensitive are also the foods that they crave the most. Desire for specific foods is also often linked to our emotional needs, force of habit, or even bodily detoxification. How then can we begin to decipher one food desire from the next?

Authors Susie Miller and Karen Knowler address this question in the book *Feel-Good Food: A Guide to Intuitive Eating*. They suggest that by giving our bodies a living food experience, we help to clear the often-confused pathways to our innate (or intuitive) knowledge of what it is we need. "As you return to the diet your body was designed for," write Miller and Knowler, "the signals start to become incredibly clear, and consequently it isn't long before you can begin to trust your instincts again." In addition to a living diet Miller and Knowler point to a path of "inner awareness," which includes looking at cultural influences and emotional needs (such as self-esteem) as well as practicing non-judgment and uninterrupted self-observation. Many people also find it helpful to receive feedback from health professionals using methods such as kinesiology or electro-dermal screening to help determine any specific food sensitivities or deficiencies.

In addition to the above-mentioned nutrient sources, other prenatal nutritional concerns for many women include getting enough calcium, zinc, and vitamin D. Calcium-rich foods include: leafy greens, legumes, tahini (sesame butter), sunflower seeds, and nuts. High amounts of zinc are found in whole grains, leafy greens, mushrooms, nuts, seeds (especially tahini), legumes, tofu, miso, wheat germ, and nutritional yeast. Vitamin D, which is better described as a hormone than a vitamin, is created by our own bodies as a result of sunlight shining onto our skin. This activates a fatty substance called ergosterol that becomes active "vitamin D" in our bloodstream and enables the absorption of calcium. "Sunlight is so effective in creating vitamin D," says Klaper, "that 15 minutes of sunlight exposure on the face and arms is all that is required to meet our daily needs." This can even be met through an open window. Vitamin D is also stored in the liver to provide us a continued supply during seasonal changes. (For pregnant women who are not able to receive adequate sunlight, however, vitamin D supplementation is advisable.)

❦ REMEDIES FOR NAUSEA

Morning sickness has also been connected to low blood sugar. In her book *Wise Woman Herbal for the Childbearing Year,* Susan Weed recommends eating small, frequent meals throughout the day as well as eating a protein-rich snack before going to sleep. Weed writes that morning sickness may also be attributed to the chemical by-products of pregnancy that can build-up in the body (she says, "Walk a mile a day to prevent this") or to the deficiency of iron or of vitamin B-6.

Other *Wise Woman* recommendations include plenty of fresh air, visualization (to get to the root of emotional aspects of the issue), and the following tea tonics sipped first thing in the morning:

1. A cup of anise or fennel-seed tea;

2. One teaspoon of apple-cider vinegar in 8 ounces of warm water;

3. A cup or two of raspberry leaf tea or an infusion each day; sucking on ice-cubes made from the infusion increases the strength of this remedy;

4. A peppermint or spearmint infusion;

5. Tablespoon doses of gingerroot tea (anytime nausea occurs, not necessarily in the morning);

6. Dehydration can also be a factor; drink plenty of water.

❦ KNOW YOUR FOOD

A word of warning: Pregnancy is the time of all times to be informed about which raw foods are edible. During my first trimester of pregnancy a well-meaning friend once served me raw elderberries in a salad. Thankfully, my body took immediate action, and I was purging miserably for an hour and a half. Every conceivable trace of the berry was ejected, and thereafter the mere thought of elderberries provoked intense nausea. It wasn't until months later that I came across a list of toxic plants that included the elderberry. Even some edible and medicinal herbs can put the unborn at risk. Check labels, ask a trusted herbalist, and if in doubt, do without!

⚜ Pre-natal Juice Boosts

I can't say enough about juicing fresh fruits and vegetables throughout pregnancy. It's such a great way to bolster nutrition for you and baby, especially for those times when you don't feel like eating for two.

Iron Woman Refresher

This combination befriended me on a day when I felt a need for additional iron. It was a day that the thought of green juice with carrot just wasn't appealing. I happened to look over at the leftover water from some raisins I'd soaked and a new recipe was born. It's light and sweet with a squeeze of vitamin C. "Did I really just drink all of those beet greens?" I thought.

> 2 small red beets, beet greens included
> Small handful parsley
> 1 lemon, wedged and peeled
> 1 cup raisin-soak water (may need to be diluted to cut
>   sweetness depending on how many raisins were used)

Chop the red beets and juice alternately with the greens and lemon to help to push them through the hopper (if not using a "green juicer"). In a large glass of ice, combine with the raisin-soak water and stir.

For more mild fruit and veggie juice ideas, see the "Kiddie Cocktails" in the "Recipes for Children" section.

Feeding Baby

Give a baby a banana and a live rabbit. I can bet you my car that every single time the baby will eat the banana and play with the rabbit.

— Harvey Diamond, *Fit for Life*

♣ Breastfeeding: Baby's First Instinct

By the twentieth week of pregnancy a baby is skilled at thumb sucking, practicing coordinated movements that will be needed later for feeding.

— Sheila Kitzinger, *Breastfeeding Your Baby*

It has been observed that like all of the other mammals, a human infant, when left to her natural instincts, will wiggle her tiny body across her mother's, locate her mother's breasts, and begin to nurse just moments after birth. A mother's body when left to its intelligence is signaled by the birth of the placenta to release hormones (prolactin and ocitocin) that stimulate the milk-creating cells of her breasts. Colostrum is already present as a perfect transitional food for the infant's first few days from the womb. Along with its nourishment, this pre-milk contains the antibodies that an infant's body cannot yet produce on its own. A laxative, it also helps to empty the baby's digestive system of meconium and excess mucus, thus preventing jaundice.

The stimulation of the suckling baby, in turn, grants gifts of its own to the mother. Her uterus is prompted to shrink back into pre-pregnancy position and her hormones are aided in re-balancing, thus helping to prevent post-partum depression.

A mother's breasts continue creating milk so long as the infant continues to nurse. The more the baby suckles, the more milk her breasts will make. Cradled in, skin-to-skin, next to his mother's heart the newborn receives his first taste of food in the context of warmth, protection, and love.

With the added insight of our food being a living system, we gain an even greater glimpse of breast milk's nurturing vitality. At body temperature mother's milk is a complete source of enzymes, hormones, essential fatty acids, vitamins, and minerals. Its proteins, fats, and carbohydrates are a proportional match for the specific needs of a growing infant.

Even more remarkable are the ways in which a mother's milk adapts as the needs of her baby change. In addition to the change from colostrum to more substantial milk, breast milk will vary at different times during the day and even throughout the duration of each feeding. When a baby comes to the breast, for example, the milk that is available first (the foremilk) is watery, and so a short nursing will satiate a baby who is simply thirsty. As he continues to suck (from the same breast) he will then receive the hind-milk, which is richer.

It is not uncommon for a breastfeeding mother to experience food cravings that are so often associated with pregnancy. A mother on a natural diet, who tunes into these bodily signals, can often see a correlation between the foods she craves and the changing nutritional needs of her child. It was when our Quinn was around six months old, for example, that my love affair with leafy greens began. This is the age when it is said that the reserve of iron an infant is born with has been depleted and an intake of dietary iron is needed. I've also witnessed major protein cravings that were followed by my daughter's hair growing like wild.

Despite the separation that takes place between mother and baby at birth, we see that in the relationship of breastfeeding, our bodies continue to operate as one system. In this holistic light many questions arise regarding our culture's practice of early infant-mother separation and breastfeeding replacements.

Infant formula has often been touted as viable nutrition to offer to our children. In the 1950s up to the 1970s it was even commonly viewed to be a superior feeding choice because it was scientific. With the new information becoming available, however, today's nutritionists now come to the unanimous consensus that breast is best. In the context of living nutrition breast milk is not only of vital essence, but its manufactured imitation is held under great suspicion.

Not only is formula lacking the countless benefits unique to mother's milk, but the very ingredients of which it is comprised raise the label reader's brow. Refined sugar, for starters, (most often in the form of corn syrup) is formula's first ingredient. Its vitamins are also synthetic, which is to say not always assimilable and often detrimental to the body.

What about supplemental feeding? Mothers throughout the ages have provided thoroughly for their babies' needs through the practice of exclusive nursing. A mother who is in good health, who is relaxed and trusting of her body's knowledge will almost always produce enough milk for her young. Some breastfeeding advocates have even proposed that the "insufficient milk syndrome" we're hearing more about now is little more than a ploy by the infant formula business to win back the dollars of breastfeeding mothers. Given the lack of integrity that some of these companies have displayed (namely in third world countries where breastfeeding is often a matter of life or death), it does raise one's suspicions. There are, however, some modern lifestyle factors, such as taking medications or eating an unnatural diet that do influence a mother's milk supply.

In addition, new mothers are often misinformed about their infants' feeding needs. Although the benefits of colostrum are well documented, for example, it is still not unheard of for medical personnel to give a newborn formula rather than to allow the exclusive nursing of the mother's pre-milk.

❧ Ways to Increase Your Milk Supply

1. Increase your intake of pure water and other nourishing fluids such as nut milks and freshly extracted juices.

2. Nurture your body with plenty of whole and living foods. Taking off the extra weight accumulated in pregnancy is a concern common to many of us, but skipping meals or pinching calories can deny you and baby vital nutrients as well as lower your milk supply. By simply breastfeeding, you help your body lose extra pounds. Replacing processed foods (even those that are labeled "low fat") with a diet rich in raw, plant-based foods also does wonders! We tend to overeat largely because our bodies are not getting what they need from heavily cooked and refined foods, and so we eat more bulk in order to make up for these nutrients. Getting enough nourishing foods to eat actually helps to maintain a healthy body weight and provides nourishment for the baby.

3. Drink teas made of the following herbs: nettles, alfalfa, red clover, comfrey, raspberry leaf, fennel, fenugreek, or caraway seeds. Midwives have long used these mild herbs to help women increase their milk flow. They offer nutritive value and are safe for the baby. Traditional Medicinals makes a "Mother's Milk Tea" that combines some of the above mentioned herbs.

4. Relaxation techniques such as massage, peaceful thoughts, stretching, and deep breathing can help you and baby bond. Stress decreases milk production so rest, relax, and be kind to yourself as much as possible. Other stress-relievers: taking a warm soak or spending time in nature (such as leisurely walks, or respites on a blanket with the baby out under a tree).

5. Think milk. The relationship between mind and body is profound. Constant fretting over whether or not we're making enough milk sends the signal "not enough milk" to the body. Visualize abundance and pass on that message.

6. Eliminate alcohol and caffeine. Like the use of other drugs, these two American favorites decrease a mother's milk production. If you're concerned about not having enough breast milk, it will serve you well to take a break from them for a while.

✤ ALTERNATIVES WHEN MOTHER'S MILK CANNOT BE GIVEN

A mother's milk is the only food that has been finely crafted by nature to meet all of an infant's changing needs. Any time this milk is replaced, it needs to be approached with greatest care. The following options are offered in order to assist in the rare occasion that a mother's milk cannot be exclusively given:

1. *Another mother's milk:* Also known as a "wet nurse" this is the original substitute for the birth mother's milk. In many parts of the world it is not uncommon for lactating women to nurse another's child during times of need. A baby is oftentimes left with an older woman, for example, such as a grandmother and other women who will breast-feed the child if needed while the birth mother works in the fields. In previous eras this was widely practiced here in the United States. Today's more clinical version of sharing breast milk is the breast milk bank. It is standard procedure in hospital banks to heat the donated breast milk to 144.5°F for thirty minutes to destroy any harmful bacteria or viruses which may be present and then to freeze it at −0.4°F or lower. As a result, the milk's enzymes as well as some of its nutriment and anti-infective properties are sacrificed. This does, however, offer an alternative to formula in cases of medical emergency. Not all hospitals have milk banks. The Human Milk Banking Association of North America (HMBANA) is another resource for locating expressed

breast milk from other local mothers (see "References, Further Reading, and Resources" section for more info).

There is also a growing interest in adoptive nursing. Although most adoptive mothers need to supplement their breast milk, an infant's suck has been known to stimulate milk flow regardless of whether or not the mother has ever had or nursed a baby before! Because the amount of milk (if any) is unpredictable, Kathleen Huggins R.N., M.S. in *Nursing Mother's Companion* recommends the use of a breast milk supplementation device, which is designed to provide supplemental milk at the same time the infant is nursing. This way, a baby can get immediate satisfaction while simultaneously receiving whatever milk the mother produces.

2. *Raw goat's milk:* The living foods diet is primarily a plant-based diet. Under some circumstances, however, you may find the occasional use of raw goat's milk beneficial. In *Pregnancy, Children and the Hallelujah Diet* (a raw-foods-dominant diet), Olin Ildol, N.D., C.N.C. offers the following raw goat's milk homemade formula, which he says has been used successfully as a breast milk alternative: ⅓ raw goat's milk, ⅓ freshly extracted carrot and celery juice (two-thirds carrot and one-third celery), ⅓ purified water. The addition of the carrot and celery juice is to "help to overcome folate deficiency of goat's milk."

Goat milk is noted for its greater similarity to human milk than cow milk and therefore its greater compatibility with our own digestion. Like breast milk, it is richer in fats than cow milk and has smaller protein molecules. Raw goat milk will keep for four days refrigerated.

Fresh, high-quality, raw goat milk is not easily accessible. However, it can be obtained from the farm directly in some states. Unfortunately, milks from your local grocer have all been heated to kill any bacteria that could be present. Making sure the goat milk is organic is important because this means that the animals have been raised without the use of drugs, hormones, and chemically treated feed. Ildol suggests also adding ½ teaspoon of Udo's Choice Perfected Oil Blend to two or three feedings daily "to help ensure adequate intake of Essential

Fatty Acids." (See also the "Superfoods and Babies" section for info on flaxseed oil and babies.)

3. *Raw almond milk:* Some nutritionists suggest the use of finely strained, organic almond milk (see the "Recipes for Children" section) as a breast milk supplement; however, it is not a complete food to be used as a replacement. Almonds are a rich source of minerals such as calcium, iron, magnesium, and phosphorus and are a source of vitamin E and B vitamins. Almonds are also noted for their especially alkalinizing properties. Breast milk (as well as other raw milks) is naturally alkaline forming, whereas formula and pasteurized milks have an acidifying effect within the body.

❧ STARTING SOLID FOODS: TAKING CUES FROM BABY

> *. . . The little child shall lead them.*
>
> — Isaiah 11:6

In a hurried, highly individualistic culture we can easily find ourselves rushing to get to the next stage of our children's development, placing added emphasis on each step of their independence from us. Meanwhile nature, it seems, has a timetable of her own—a rhythmic cycle to which the closer we remain in sync, the greater our experience of overall health and well-being will be. Our very bodies are nature after all, ticking right along with the greater biological clock of the cosmos.

Not altogether comfortable with the notion of breastfeeding to begin with, modern-day culture has hastened the transition from breast milk to solid foods. A century ago babies commonly received their first solid foods sometime around their first birthday. When commercial "baby foods" first hit the shelves, however, feeding them to infants of only a few weeks in age became en vogue. Nowadays parents are being advised to wait on solids until at least the fourth month. The American Academy of Pediatrics and the World Health Organization both recommend that babies be exclusively breastfed for their first six months of life. Some parents feel most comfortable delaying solids until the later months of their babies' first year, particularly if there is a history of food allergies in the family. The more that we pause to observe our natural rhythms, the more insight we gain as to the importance of following a baby's lead for indications of her readiness for solids.

One reason to do this is that baby's digestive system needs time to mature. The absence of teeth not only indicates babies' inability to chew adult foods, but it's also a sign that their bodies are not yet fully prepared for the digestion of solids. Pepsin and gastric acid, which assist in the digestion of protein, are secreted at birth and build up to sufficient amounts over the next four months. Pancreatic enzymes (such as amylase, maltase, somaltase, and sucrase) reach adult levels for the digestion of starches sometime around baby's sixth month, whereas lipase and bile salts, aiding the digestion of fats, need six to nine months to reach adult levels.

In addition, a younger baby's digestive tract is more porous than one that has matured. This "open gut" benefits the exclusively breastfed baby by allowing his mother's antibodies to pass into his own bloodstream. Until the baby's gut has "closed" (usually between four and six months), however, the protein molecules of other foods can also leak into the bloodstream. This is the believed cause of allergic reactions to solid food in young infants.

❧ Signs of Readiness

Because the rate of growth and development can vary so greatly from one child to the next, taking cues from baby gives a better idea of what his individual needs may be. As we have seen, social trends don't always match up with the bodily timing of our children. Here are some indications that your baby may be ready for more than breast milk in his diet: the presence of teeth; the absence of the protrusion reflex (baby can receive solids without automatically spitting them out); the ability to turn his head away to indicate when he's had enough to eat;

baby shows an interest in food, such as reaching for what you're eating; baby cries or otherwise seems hungry just after nursing; or baby begins to chew on the breasts.

❦ INNATE CURIOSITY
AND THE PERIOD OF NUTRITIONAL ABSORBENCY

The child is endowed with an inner power that can guide us to a more luminous future.

— Maria Montessori

As baby grows older and his body is more prepared for solids, his natural curiosity about these foods also grows. Able to sit on his own now, he reaches for objects to look at, to handle, and to taste. The objects that he sees you putting into your mouth are now of particular interest. Observing the colors, shapes, and smells, he watches attentively to your chewing and swallowing. He may salivate, smack his own lips, reach for your spoon, or otherwise appear to ask you for a try.

As instinct first led baby to suckle the breast, instinct now directs the observation of her parents, the primary guides in her exploration of what it is that we humans eat. In the book *Biomimicry: Innovations Inspired by Nature*, Janine M. Benyus refers to these early feeding lessons among other mammals. "With primates (and many other animals, such as elephants)," she says, "the learning begins with mom. Infants will peer and poke into their mother's mouth to smell and taste what she is eating and after a while they build a chemical profile of what's good."

It has also been noted that from birth to approximately age seven, children absorb and retain an extraordinarily large part of what is presented to them. World-renowned childhood educator, Maria Montessori, referred to this as the "absorbent mind" and tailored her teaching methods to accommodate these special capabilities. Some Montessori teachers, for example, use what are called "bit libraries" (as in

69

bits of information). A bit library for babies might consist of series of eight-by-eleven-inch pictures of birds, whales, or anything else that is deemed as desirable knowledge for kids to have later on.

If a mother has a bit set depicting, for instance, a group of musical instruments, then she will hold each picture up in front of the child and simultaneously say the name of the instrument. Only a few seconds are spent on each picture, much like flash cards. In this way babies experience a lot of learning in a few minutes, a couple of times a day; it is retained for future use—and they eat it up!

Similarly, we can quite naturally introduce small "bits" of quality foods to our little ones. While breastfeeding continues to provide the primary source of nutrition, we can greet our babies' curiosities (and their absorbent minds) with daily opportunities to explore what we are up to. In a culture that places baby in a separate high chair and then offers him food by the jar, we have created limited access to the discovery of what the grown-ups eat.

Finding opportunities to feed this learning need not be formalized or complex. With my own daughter, I found that during meal preparations was a good time to include her in my activities. While I sliced one carrot, I'd offer another to teethe on. When I cut open a cucumber, I'd show her the inside and offer a lick. On a blanket, she would play with measuring spoons, a lemon, or a cauliflower head, and I'd tell her their names. Obviously it's important to be watchful of any potential choking hazards. Once a baby's teeth start coming in, he can bite off pieces of hard fruits and veggies that he cannot yet chew.

As we began to introduce new foods to Quinn, nothing felt more natural and magical to me than when we were in a garden. Before many words hold meaning, this setting provides baby a holistic experience of the new foods she is discovering. What a gift it is for a child to know the melon vine or the fig tree as being as much a part of mealtime as the bib, the bowl, or the spoon. Our children absorb these experiences like little sponges, and these memories become frames of reference for their future.

❧ STARTER FOODS THAT DON'T REQUIRE COOKING

*Fresh raw fruit is the ideal food to lead the transition while
continuing with nursing.*

> — Olin Ildol, N.D., C.N.C., *Pregnancy, Children,
> and the Hallelujah Diet*

Here in the U.S., it is somewhat standard for babies to be offered
instant rice cereal for their first taste of solid foods. This has become
the common recommendation not necessarily because rice cereal is
the best thing for infants, but because rice is considered one of the least
likely foods to trigger allergic reactions, and a product can therefore be
made from it that is deemed safe to give to all babies. Their increased
need for dietary iron is another reason why this iron-enriched cereal
is often recommended for the four-to-six-month-old baby. As we have
discussed earlier, however, vitamins and minerals that are synthetic are
less than optimal for growing bodies. The breastfed baby does receive
some iron from mother's milk. As baby grows and begins teething, a
mother who is nursing exclusively may want to add more iron-rich
foods such as fresh leafy greens, spirulina, kelp, dried fruit, and whole
grains to her own diet. Also read on for information on the use of
spirulina and other greens in your homemade baby foods.

Despite the commercial influences on modern nutrition, more and
more parents are seeking alternatives to the nutrient-stripped, cooked,
and processed baby food-products. Looking to the natural world, many
have found soft, mashable fruits such as avocado, banana, or watermelon to be choice, first foods for introducing their babies to solids.
These are naturally milder and easier to digest than tougher foods that
need to be cooked and/or blended before they can be offered to babies.
As dietary consultant Rita Romano points out in *Dining in the Raw*,
"Raw fruit is considered a predigested food in its own right. It contains
its own digestive enzymes and passes through to the intestines more

quickly than most other foods. Melons," she says, "are the most easily digested of all foods and are best eaten alone or with other melons." (We found this to be true with our baby's early feedings of watermelon. Because melon is digested more quickly than breast milk, indigestion can result when the two foods are mixed in the stomach. When we started timing the feeding of melon one-half to one hour before or after a meal of breast milk, the problem was eliminated.)

Not only is fresh fruit easily digested, but also when fully ripened (their most nutritious and desirable state) most fruits have an alkaline forming effect on the body, as opposed to the acidifying effect that results from eating cooked grains.

Like rice, however, bananas can be somewhat constipating when they are new to baby or when consumed in large amounts. It is best, therefore, to start baby out with very small portions in the beginning and see how he does with it.

Other soft, mashable fruits include papaya, pears, peaches, nectarines, and apricots (skins and seeds removed). Unless pureed, these fruits are not as smooth in texture as bananas or avocados. When simply mashed, they make a better second-step food for when baby has had some practice with solids and is starting to prefer foods that are lumpier in texture. Fresh figs and persimmons are two of my soft-fruit favorites. When very ripe, the tops can be opened with a knife and the supple flesh simply spooned out. It's as convenient as jarred baby food, only you can eat or compost the "jar." Fresh figs that have ripened well before harvest are hard to come by, however, unless they grow in your area. Because the seeds create some roughage, figs are best offered after baby's digestive system has had some exposure to solids. The flesh of raw apples can be scraped with a spoon as well.

Naturally soft tomatoes, berries, and other citrus fruits are too acidic for younger babies' digestive systems. Because they are a leading allergen for babies, the general recommendation is to wait on citrus foods until baby is a year old (and then use somewhat moderately).

❧ BABY BLENDS

Some parents feel most comfortable using soft fruits only, rather than pureeing other foods that baby would not otherwise be able to naturally eat. The rationale is that by blending harder solids for a baby one potentially introduces adult foods into an infant digestive system, a system that might not yet be equipped to process such foods. When I began my own search for nature's best baby food, I found myself pondering what our earliest ancestors might have done in order to feed their young, particularly when softer fruits were scarce or out of season. What were their natural instincts and ingenuities before the days of instant mixes, ovens, or baby food grinders? I thought of the various bird species and of our fellow mammal the whale, and how they predigest food for their babies until they've developed the ability to fully digest them on their own. I theorized that once upon a time, perhaps, it had come just as naturally for us to also chew-up roots, seeds, and greens before offering them to our little ones. Perhaps this practice was lost over time much the same way that our instinct to breastfeed is now threatened by modern notion and invention.

As it turns out, pre-mastication (or pre-chewing) is in fact practiced in various cultures. The book *Babies Celebrated* features a photo of a mother passing food directly from her own mouth into her baby's mouth. Water is also sometimes given in this way. Paul Pitchford mentions the pre-chewing of food for babies in *Healing with Whole Foods: Asian Traditions and Modern Nutrition*. He recommends the practice stating that the enzymes in the adult saliva are made available to the infant in this way, thus helping to make the food more easily digested.

I find a sense of satisfaction in getting in touch with my primitive side, as well as in sticking out a defiant tongue to my early years in table manner training, but I must admit that as a product of my environment my first instinct has been to employ my blender, grater, or juicer, when creating my own baby foods at home. I've found my appliances especially helpful when preparing meals for the whole family. In the following recipes, for example, you will find baby purees that can also double as raw soups, smoothies, or sauces for older children and/or grown-ups.

For those who choose to make homemade baby blends, it is important to note that there are foods to avoid for the younger baby (see "Food Introduction Guide"). These include raw honey, citrus, strong spices, and gas-producing vegetables (beans, garlic, onion, broccoli, etc.). With the exception of soaked almonds, nuts also tend to provoke allergic reaction when introduced too soon. In *Pregnancy, Children and the Vegan Diet*, Michael Klaper, M.D. suggests the age of one year for the introduction of nuts and nut butters. Families with food allergies may do well to delay nuts until later.

Salt and refined sugars are other ingredients best left out of a baby's first foods. Too much salt can put strain on an infant's young kidneys and even small amounts of refined sugar suppress the immune system. Pitchford's salt recommendation is none before ten months of age and then to start adding one grain at a time. A baby easily meets her bodily requirement of salt from the fruits, veggies, and small amounts of sea vegetables in her diet. (Regular table salt, which is not considered healthful, can be easily replaced with sea salt or Celtic salt.) Refined sugar is best avoided altogether. Stevia, agave nectar, fresh fruit/juice, and reconstituted dried fruit are all excellent raw food replacements.

❧ Nut Milks and Diluted Juices

Well-strained, raw almond milk as well as diluted juices from milder fruits and vegetables can also be offered as beginner foods. Potent cleansers such as gingerroot, beets, or wheat grass juice are best introduced after baby is more established on solids and given in small amounts. Veggies from the allium family (onions, garlic, shallots, and leeks) as well as the brasicas (cabbage, cauliflower, brussels sprouts, broccoli, and kale) tend to be gaseous and therefore are best left out of baby cocktails as well.

When making almond milk, soak the almonds overnight or for eight to twelve hours ahead of time. This deactivates the growth inhibitor hormones that render them less digestible. Sprouting nuts in this way also gives them a nutritional boost. Other nuts and seeds can also be soaked and blended into milks in this way, but it is the recommendation to introduce these later on. If you live in a tropical area, water from fresh young coconuts is another mild and nourishing first fluid. Buying them imported, however, can be somewhat questionable, as the young coconuts may have been chemically treated in order to preserve them long enough to travel overseas.

⚜ SUPERFOODS AND BABIES

In a budding era of better living through nutrition, new and special foods have been gaining public attention for their unique and health-promoting qualities. Endowed with a reserve of nutrients that soars above other whole food sources, these newly famed foods such as flaxseeds, spirulina, and sprouts are often nicknamed "superfoods." As invaluable to our health as these superfoods are, information on their use with young children is still just coming out. As time goes on we will know much more. In the meantime, however, here are some specifics on a few of these foods to help with decision-making on how to best use them in your family's diet.

Breast milk: It bears repeating, when it comes to superfoods, mama's milk tops them all! The breast milk of a healthy mother has everything needed to grow her baby. Mama's milk can even be dropped into her infant's eyes to treat a case of pinkeye. No matter how amazing other superfoods may be (and despite what any advertisers may claim) the following high-nutrition foods are not suitable replacements for breast milk. (Attempting to use them as such is not only unnatural but puts an infant's health at serious risk.)

Flaxseed oil: The little flaxseed has been making a big name for itself on account of the omega-3 fatty acids found in its oils. As Ruth Yaron points out in *Super Baby Food*, flaxseed oil is superior to fish oils (also noted for their essential fatty acids) not only in content (and I would add flavor), but also because it is free of the mercury and lead now commonly found in fish due to polluted waters.

The best way for baby to receive the benefits of flaxseed oil is through mother's milk. When flaxseed oil is consumed by the mother, it not only passes on to baby, but the DHA (decosahexamine acid) is converted to its easily metabolized form, omega-3. Breast milk is a naturally rich source of Essential Fatty Acids (EFAs) so long as the mother is getting them in her own diet. Other foods containing omega-3's are walnuts, canola oil, olive oil, alfalfa sprouts, soybeans, and spinach. Avoiding trans-fatty acids such as in hydrogenated oils (in margarines and other processed foods) is also key. When consumed by the mother, these harmful fats are also passed on to baby through her breast milk. Associated with a number of health problems, trans-fats prohibit the metabolism of good fats (EFAs) and therefore interfere with their benefits to mother and child.

So essential are omega-3 fatty acids that some nutritionists now recommend their supplementation for non-breastfeeding infants. In *Super Immunity for Kids*, Dr. Leo Galland suggests one teaspoon of flaxseed oil per day be added to a baby's bottle. This is best spread out into smaller doses throughout the day, because some babies have trouble converting the DHA in the oil to omega-3 fatty acid. In the article, "Flaxseed Oil: Putting It to Good Use," Doh Driver recommends no more than one-eighth-teaspoon flaxseed oil be mixed into a younger baby's serving of food.

Excess oil can be a laxative and produce acid in the body. The general recommended dosage for children (according to the above mentioned article) is as follows:

20–30 lb babies and toddlers: ¼ to ½ teaspoon;
30–50 lb children: 1 teaspoon;

50–75 lb children: 2 teaspoons;

75–100 lb children: 1 tablespoon.

Babies can also receive the benefits of flaxseed oil (food grade) when it is massaged into their skin.

Once your baby is established on eating solids, freshly ground flaxseeds can be sprinkled into his food as well. This gives baby the benefits of the oils in less concentrated amounts and ensures a higher quality of freshness.

When released from the seed, flaxseed oil is highly perishable. This is why it is sold in dark-colored bottles and kept refrigerated (continue to store it in this way). To ensure freshness, check expiration dates and taste-test oils before use (flaxseed oil usually has a buttery, nutty flavor). If using freshly ground flaxseeds, grind only what will be used that day (in an electric coffee grinder) and refrigerate the ground seeds in a sealed container, if not used immediately. I also recommend using whole flaxseeds only when making dehydrated-flaxseed goods. On more than one occasion, I've experienced indigestion from rancid oils after having followed recipes that had called for ground or blended flaxseeds before dehydrating.

Micro-algae—spirulina and chlorella: Spirulina is heralded the richest source of organic protein in the vegetable kingdom, containing three times the protein found in beef. Because of its concentrated nutrition, spirulina has been used to treat infant malnutrition, both in Mexico and in China. In *Healing with Whole Foods: Asian Traditions and Modern Nutrition*, Paul Pitchford makes note of its particularly high levels of fatty acids, GLA, and omega-3-linolenic acid. He says, "GLA is important for growth and development and is found most abundantly in mother's milk; spirulina is the next-highest-whole-food source." In his practice he often recommends spirulina "for people who've never breastfed in order to foster the hormonal and mental development that may never have occurred because of the lack of proper nutrition in infancy."

Chlorella micro-algae is similar to spirulina in its nutrient profile and usage. In Pitchford's experience treating malnourishment, he finds it to be better for the extremely weak and frail child because it is "a little less cooling and cleansing."

For babies under one year Pitchford suggests a dosage of one-half teaspoon of spirulina or one-fourth teaspoon chlorella up to twice a day. These doses are recommended for malnourishment cases; however, micro-algae is also an appropriate food-source for children in good health. Once baby is established eating fruits, you may want to begin adding a little to his mashed or blended fruits.

Sprouts: Grain, nut, seed, or bean sprouts contain more live enzymes and energy than any other food. These wee baby plants abound in protein, chlorophyll (green sprouts), vitamins, minerals, and amino acids. Each type of sprout has its own distinctive super powers, so eating a wide variety gives all the powers they have to offer. Sunflower seed sprouts, for example, are a rich source of highly digestible protein, whereas sesame seed sprouts are noted for their bio-available calcium. Buckwheat greens give us lecithin; fenugreek supports our lymphatic system; wheat grass purifies the blood and the liver; and alfalfa sprouts aid our digestion. Have you heard about sulfurophane, the antioxidant that puts broccoli on all the anti-cancer food lists? Broccoli sprouts have been found to contain fifty times more of this than found in mature broccoli. New research also indicates that peanut sprouts might reduce unhealthy cholesterol.

With their tremendous health benefits and very simple cultivation, it's no wonder why sprouts have been grown by numerous civilizations for over 5,000 years. Sprouting nuts, beans, seeds, and grains in order to spark the life of these otherwise dormant staples has always been a major component of the living-foods diet. Some nutritionists suggest blending green sprouts in water for the six-month-old baby, while others recommend waiting on the feeding of all sprouts until ten to twelve months. Utilize sprouts as you feel most comfortable. I personally found it helpful to categorize the different varieties when making decisions on which sprouts to introduce at what time:

1. *Milder sprouts and micro-greens:* These are seeds that have been sprouted until they bear little greens leaves. Buckwheat, sunflower, flax, chia, alfalfa, and clover are milder varieties than the brassicas and spicy sprouts. Suggested age: six months and up, if blended in water or diluted juices.

2. *Brassicas and spicy sprouts:* These include broccoli, cabbage, onion, garlic, mustard, and radish. Suggested age: one year and up.

3. *Soaked seeds:* Sometimes referred to as "soaks" rather than "sprouts," these are seeds soaked before usage but not fully sprouted into micro-greens. Sesame, sunflower, buckwheat, pumpkin, and flax are commonly used this way in raw-food preparation. Suggested age: eight months on up, used in seed milks, soups, and other baby blends.

4. *Soaked nuts:* Used much the same way as the above seed "soaks," these nuts include soaked almonds, walnuts, pecans, brazil nuts, macadamias, pine nuts, and hazelnuts. Suggested age: one year on up for all nuts except for almonds, which can be used for almond milk starting at the age of six months or even as a breast milk supplement.

5. *Legumes:* Mung beans, peas, chickpeas, lentils, and adzuki beans are common eatable legume sprouts. The sprouting of legumes renders them more digestible than does cooking them. However, some people still have difficulty with them and omit legumes completely from their raw-foods diet. We enjoy using them for the added variety of flavors and nutrition. Suggested age: one year on up.

6. *Sprouted grains:* Cereal grains such as wheat, quinoa, spelt, amaranth, kamut, barley, rye, and oats can be sprouted for raw cereals, salads, and dehydrated breads. These are simply soaked over-

night, or sprouted, just until small "tails" appear. Suggested age: ten months on up for blended cereals; ages fourteen to eighteen months on up for breads.

7. *Grasses:* These are grains that have been sprouted in soil in order to reap the benefits of their greens. Many cereal grains can be sprouted into grass and then juiced, or juiced, and dehydrated. Wheat grass juice and barley green are widely used this way for their cleansing and energizing properties. Although freshly extracted, green juice is more potent, powdered forms may be most practical for day-to-day use or when traveling. Dehydrated barley green can be added to pureed baby foods or mixed into fruit juice or water. When shopping for a green powder, you will want to ensure that the juice is organic and was processed at low temperatures to preserve the natural enzymes. Suggested age: six months on up for fresh grasses blended in water or other diluted juices, gradually working up to freshly extracted juices diluted with 50% or more purified water.

☙ FOOD INTRODUCTION GUIDE

Age-appropriate baby-food charts are popular with a number of parents. They provide lists of specific food items and indicate which may be compatible with baby's digestion at what particular month of age. For a more detailed chart (distinctively for raw foods) look for the newly released book *Rainbow Green Live-Food Cuisine* by Gabriel Cousens, M.D. Ruth Yaron's extensive book *Super Baby Foods* also features a food chart that is inclusive of some raw foods.

After referencing a number of charts from different books and finding much discrepancy between their recommendations, I've personally abandoned strict adherence to any one particular chart. The following are general recommendations, however, that I've found to be common to various introductory food guides. Use according to your individual needs.

Approximate Age	Food
Birth through 18–24 months+	Breast milk
6 months+	Almond mild
	Freshly extracted juices: Dilute with 50% or more purified water. Start with mild fruits (such as melon), followed by mild veggie juices (such as carrot/celery, carrot/lettuce)
	Mashed/pureed raw fruits: Start with mono, sweet fruits (melon, banana, persimmon, sapote) and/or non-sweets (cucumber, avocado). Gradually follow with sub-acids (apple, papaya, pears, apricots, nectarines, peaches, mangos, plums, guava, cherries, etc.)
	Dried fruit: Soak 8–12 hours then puree with water/soak water
8 months+	Raw vegetables soups/purees: Use mild veggies (lettuce, celery, parsley, jicama, carrots, snow peas, sweet corn, etc.)
	Pureed/mashed steamed veggies
	Seed milks
	Tahini (sesame butter) and other ground/blended seeds (flax, pumpkin, sunflower, chia, hemp, etc.)
10 months+	Starchy foods: Pureed cereals from sprouted wild rice, buckwheat, or whole grains (oats, barley, quinoa, millet, etc.)
	Cooked grains/potatoes
1 year+	Acid fruits: citrus, tomatoes, berries, etc.
	Raw honey
	Fermented foods
	High protein foods:
	Nut butters (almond, macadamia)
	Most other nuts (ground/soaked and blended): walnuts, pecans, pine nuts, hazelnuts, etc.
	Legumes (moderate use): chickpeas, mung beans, lentils, dried peas, etc.
14–18 months+	Breads (dehydrated/baked)
	Pasta
	Family meals

❧ RECIPES FOR BABY

Fruit Mash

For an easy to make baby food, take any one of the following soft fruits, remove any skins, stones, or tough/stringy fibers and mash it with a fork until smooth in consistency: avocado, banana, persimmon, papaya, pear, apricot, nectarine, peach, mango, plum, or fig.

Cherry-Banana-Peach Sauce

Yields 2 adult servings and 1 baby-sized serving.

    2 bananas, peeled and chopped
    2 peaches, pitted and chopped
    2 cups sweet cherries, halved (stones removed)
    2 peaches, pitted and sliced

In a blender or food processor, blend together the bananas, 2 chopped peaches and 1 cup of the halved sweet cherries. (If using a blender, you may have to add very small amounts of water to allow the blades to turn.) Pour out a serving for baby and set aside. For the grown-up and/or older child serve the cherry-banana-peach sauce over the remaining sliced peaches and sweet cherry halves.

Variation: When baby has graduated to berries, substitute blueberries for cherries.

Carrot-Banana Smoothie

Yields 1 adult and 1 baby-sized serving.

1½ cup fresh carrot juice
1 frozen banana, broken into pieces
¼ cup freshly grated carrot

In a blender, puree the above ingredients until smooth (adding more liquid to thin). Ice-cold foods can be especially helpful for soothing sore, teething gums. Also refer to the "Recipes for Children" section for additional frozen treats.

Variation: Replace banana with frozen mango chunks.

Waldorf Pudding

Yields 2 adult servings and 1 baby-sized serving.

1 banana, peeled and chopped
1 avocado, peeled, pitted, and chopped
1 apple, cored and chopped
1 apple
¼ cup raisins, soaked until softened (at least 3 hours)
⅓ cup walnuts

In a food processor or blender, blend together the banana, avocado, and one of the apples, adding just enough raisin-soak water to achieve a smooth yet thick consistency. Pour pudding into serving cups and chill. Just before serving, chop the second apple and drop into the adult servings along with the raisins and walnuts. A fresh sprig of mint also makes a pretty garnish.

Pear – Spirulina

Yields 1 baby-sized serving.

½ pear
¼ teaspoon spirulina

Finely grate the ½ pear. Mix in spirulina.

Variation: Substitute chlorella for spirulina or apple for the pear.

Banana – Chlorella

Yields 1 baby-sized serving.

½ banana, peeled
¼ teaspoon chlorella

Mash banana with a fork and mix in chlorella.

Variation: Substitute spirilina for chlorella.

Avocado-Spirulina-Kelp Spread

Yields 1 baby-sized serving.

½ avocado
¼ teaspoon kelp
¼ teaspoon spirulina flakes

Mash avocado and mix in kelp and spirulina. Sample a little yourself. If you like it as much as baby does, make some extra to spread on your crackers or celery sticks.

Apple with Green Juice

Yields 1 baby-sized serving.

1 ounce green juice
½ apple

In a juicer, make yourself a green juice (example: cucumber-celery-kale), reserving 1 ounce for the baby blend. For a finer sauce for the younger baby: peel and chop the apple and process it along with the 1 ounce green juice in a baby-food grinder, mini food processor, or blender until it is smooth in texture. The apple can also be sauced by running it through a Champion juicer using the blank screen. For the older baby the apple can be finely grated using a manual grater. Next, stir in the 1 ounce green juice by hand.

Apple-Carrot Salad with Raisin Sauce

Yields 1 baby-sized serving.

½ apple
½ small carrot
1–2 tablespoon raisin-soak water

Finely grate apple and carrot. Add raisin-soak water and mix.

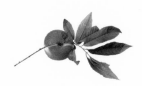

Cucumber-Apple Sauce

Yields 1 baby-sized serving.

½ apple
½ small cucumber

Method 1: For the solid-food beginner, peel both the apple and cucumber and remove any seeds (as these may cause gagging). Next chop both "fruits" and puree together in a blender or baby-food grinder adding small amounts of water or apple juice to achieve a smooth consistency.

Method 2: For the experienced solid-food eater peels and cucumber seeds are not problematic unless the produce has been waxed and/or chemically treated. If the cucumber is not peeled, it can be finely grated along with the apple, rather than pureed. Grate your desired amount and mix the two sauces together. The combination has a refreshing, mildly sweet flavor.

Banana-Tahini Pudding

Banana and tahini make a sweet and creamy combination. Mash the amount of banana you desire with ½-part raw tahini.

Sunflower Cereal

Yields 1 baby-sized serving.

¼ cup sunflower seeds, soaked for 8–12 hours
½ Bosc pear, chopped
Dash of cinnamon (optional)

After soaking the sunflower seeds, drain and discard the soak water. Puree the soaked seeds with the chopped pear, adding just enough water/fruit juice/or dried-fruit-soak water to blend into a smooth consistency. Sprinkle with cinnamon.

Variation: Substitute fresh peach or apple for the pear.

Carrot-Apricot Puree

Yields 1 baby-sized serving.

½ medium sized carrot, chopped
3 dried apricots, soaked for 8–12 hours in
½ cup water

Puree carrot, apricots, and soak water until all the chunks are gone and the mixture has reached a smooth consistency. Add more water to thin as needed.

Apple-Celery-Parsley Soup

Yields 1 adult and 1 baby-sized serving.

1 apple, cored
1 stalk celery
Handful of fresh parsley
Juice of ½ lemon*
½ cup date-soak water (or fruit juice)

Puree together and serve.

Sugarplum-Spice Soup

Yields 1 adult and 1 baby-sized serving.

3 fresh plums, pitted
½ teaspoon cinnamon
1 thin sliver of fresh gingerroot
2–4 pieces soaked dried fruit of your choice (dried apricots
    and/or prunes are nice)
½–1 cup rosehip tea (see notation below)**

Blend all the ingredients together until the mixture is a soupy consistency, adding more liquids to thin.

---

*If baby is not eating citrus yet, leave out the lemon juice when blending the whole batch and simply add it to your own after you've set a portion for baby aside. Otherwise, puree all ingredients together, adding extra liquids if needed.

**To make the rosehip tea, soak 1 teaspoon dried rosehips (or one tea bag) in 1 cup purified water overnight in the refrigerator. When the tea is infused, strain and discard the tea leaves.

Apricot-Almond Soup

Yields 1 adult and 1 baby-sized serving.

4 fresh apricots, pitted and chopped
½ cup almonds, soaked for 8–24 hours and skins removed*
2 dried apricots, soaked for 8–12 hours in ½ cup water

Blend together the fresh apricots, almonds, dried apricots, and apricot-soak water (discard the water from soaking the almonds). Add just enough water to thin, if desired.

Apple-Squash Pie

This recipe makes dessert for everyone.

10 apples cored, peeled and cut into chunks
1½ cups butternut squash, peeled, seeded and cut into chunks
2 cups dates, pitted
2 teaspoons ground cinnamon
2 tablespoons ground psyllium seed

Using a heavy-duty juicer is a bit of a production for just a few spoonfuls of baby food. Using the blank screen on your Champion (or other power juicer) process the apple, squash, and dates alternately. (If you desire less sweetness for baby, use less dates for his portion.) Stir thoroughly. Set baby's portion aside. Then, add the remaining ingredients and stir thoroughly again. Pour into your favorite piecrust (I recommend a simple, raw, almond-raisin crust) and chill until set.

---

*Almonds are more easily digested when the skins are removed—the skins are easier to peel after they've soaked for two days (the soak water needs to be changed daily for freshness). Another method for loosening peels is to pour very hot water over the soaked almonds and to then drain them right away.

Cupid's Soup

Yields 1 adult and 1 baby-sized serving.

1 large apple, cored and diced
½ small red beet, scrubbed and diced
½ lemon, peeled and seeds removed
Thin sliver fresh gingerroot
½ teaspoon cinnamon
¼ teaspoon allspice
4 dates, soaked 8–12 hours in
½ cup water

Puree all the ingredients together (including fruit-soak water), adding small amounts of extra liquid if needed.

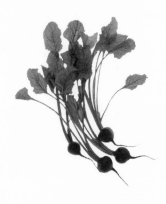

Jicama-Pear Sauce

Yields 2 adult and 1 baby-sized serving.

  1 cup chopped jicama
  2 cups chopped pear
  3–5 dates, soaked (at least one hour) in ½ cup water
  ½ cup date-soak water
  Juice of 2–4 limes
  1 teaspoon lime zest
  1-inch slice gingerroot
  2 lime wedges (for garnish)

Put jicama, pear, pitted dates, and date-soak water in blender and puree, adding more water if needed. Pour out portion for the younger baby and set aside. Add lime juice, zest, and ginger to the remaining sauce in the blender and puree again. Pour adult servings into margarita glasses (or regular drinking glasses) over crushed ice. Rub the lime wedge around the rim of the glass before attaching to the rim as a garnish. Serve sauce to baby "as is" or also over crushed ice (remove any large ice chunks).

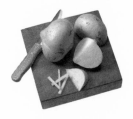

Pineapple-Lettuce-Cilantro Soup

Yields 1 adult and 1 baby-sized serving.

½ fresh pineapple, pared and chopped*
2 large romaine lettuce leaves (or 3 small leaves), torn into
    pieces
¼ cup cilantro, loosely packed
¼ cup fruit juice, water, or soak water from dried fruit

Grown-up extras:

Juice from ½ lime
½ cup mixture of halved green grapes and fresh pineapple
    chunks

In a blender combine all of the ingredients except the grown-up extras
and puree until smooth. Pour out a serving for baby and set aside. Add
lime juice to the soup in the blender and blend for just a few seconds.
Pour adult serving into a soup bowl and spoon in the remaining extras.
Serve at room temperature or chilled.

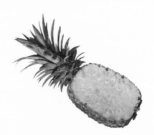

---

*Although pineapple is considered an acid fruit, it does not have the same
reputation that citrus, tomatoes, and berries have for causing an allergic
reaction. It is therefore commonly offered to babies before the age of one
year. We recommend introducing pineapple after baby is well established
on the milder fruits.

Summer Sweet-Corn Chowder

Yields 2 adult and 1 baby-sized serving.

3 ears raw sweet corn
½ large cucumber, peeled and diced
1 tablespoon nutritional yeast flakes
1 tablespoon flax seed oil/cold-pressed olive oil
1 teaspoon dried oregano
2 teaspoons ground cumin
1 teaspoon dehydrated onion powder (optional)
½ cup water

Grown-up extras:

2 tsp. miso, thinned with
2 tablespoons water
pinch of cayenne pepper
1 teaspoon garlic powder
1 cup mixture of the following minced veggies:
    red bell pepper, celery, parsley, onion

Cut the corn off the cobs, setting aside the kernels from one of the cobs. Put the remaining corn and all other ingredients except the grown-up extras into the blender and blend until smooth, adding small amounts of additional water as needed. Pour soup puree into bowls. Stir the grown-up extras into the adult servings as well as the reserved corn (from one ear). Serve at room temperature or chilled.

Variation: To serve as a "creamed corn" side dish rather than as a chowder, add additional freshly cut corn and more minced veggies.

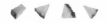

Peas Porridge Cold
(Creamy almond, fresh pea soup w/mint)

Yields 2 adult servings and 1 baby-sized serving.

2 cups thick almond milk
1 cup fresh or frozen and thawed, shelled sugar snap peas
1 medium cucumber, peeled, seeded, and chopped
Sprig of mint

Grown-up extras:

½ cup fresh, shelled, sugar snap peas
Juice of one lemon wedge
Celtic salt and cracked pepper to taste
A few small mint leaves, julienne

Combine all of the ingredients except the grown-up extras in a blender and puree until smooth. Pour into serving bowls and use the extras as garnishes for adults.

Variation: Substitute fresh dill for the mint.

Sweet Red-Pepper Soup

Yields 1 adult and 1 baby-sized serving.

1 red bell pepper, chopped
2 tablespoons pine nuts, soaked for 8–12 hours
½ teaspoon mild miso
1 stalk celery
Handful of parsley
½ cup water
Dehydrated onion flakes to taste

Puree together and serve.

Creamy Carrot-Veggie Soup

Yields 4 servings, plus 1 for baby

1 cup almonds, soaked and skins removed*
1 cucumber, peeled and cubed (seeds included)
2 cups fresh celery-carrot-lettuce juice
1 cup carrot, steamed until tender and chopped
½ red or yellow bell pepper, chopped (optional)
3 sprigs parsley or ¼ cup spinach or other mild fresh greens
1 teaspoon fresh mild miso

Grown-up seasonings:

1–2 cloves roasted garlic, ½ teaspoon garlic powder, and/or ½ teaspoon mild curry powder

Blend together all the ingredients except the grown-up seasonings.
Set baby's aside and then blend the stronger seasonings for the adult
servings.

Variation: For beet borscht, replace steamed carrots with steamed red
beets and garnish adult bowls with thin strips of raw green cabbage.

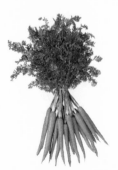

---

*Peeling the almonds contributes to the soup's smooth texture and creami-
ness. This meditative process (it's repetitive and it slows you down) can
be made easier by blanching the soaked almonds first with very hot water.
Peeling almonds can be a fun job for small-handed kitchen help.

Baby Spinach-Guacamole Dip

2 cups loosely packed baby spinach or large spinach leaves,
  chopped
4–5 avocados

For grown-ups:

½ teaspoon Mexican seasoning
½ teaspoon ground cumin
½ teaspoon sea salt or Braggs Aminos
2 tablespoons minced chives or fresh sweet onion (optional)

Wash spinach thoroughly and dry on a clean towel. Blend with avocados in a food processor (using the s-blade) until smooth or through
a Champion juicer (using the blank screen). Set aside baby's serving
and season with powdered kelp. Add the grown-up ingredients to the
remaining avocado-spinach mixture. Pulse it all together in the food
processor once more or simply stir together with a spoon.

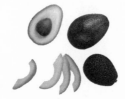

Toddler Foods

It is happy talent to know how to play.

— Ralph Waldo Emerson

*Laughter aids digestion, fosters fellowship,
and feeds the soul.*

— Peggy Jenkins, Ph.D., *The Joyful Child*

❧ CONTINUED BREASTFEEDING
MAKING PEACE WITH CULTURE CLASH

Please Mommy, can I nurse again? 'Cuz I'm really nursty.

— Quinn, age 2 ½

The wisdom that forms a tiny fetus and that leads a baby to first suckle the breast, continues to guide our children as they develop, learn, and grow. This wisdom can be witnessed with each developmental milestone, weaning being no exception. As solid foods become a part of baby's diet, his desire to nurse will naturally decrease. To their mother's surprise, some babies will even initiate full days of a "nursing strike" or weaning as early as 12 months in age. As our babies grow and find that their ability to meet their own needs is also growing, they naturally begin to explore their independence from us. They begin to feed themselves, walk, communicate through words, use the potty, and dress themselves. As children develop these new ways of meeting their needs, the old ways that served them as infants are naturally set aside.

Following a child's initiation to wean is often referred to as "natural weaning." But what if one's baby eats a variety of solids, walks, and speaks, yet still does not show interest in weaning? What if a child now has independence from diapers and is even attempting to dress herself, yet she still desires her mother's breast? Has something gone awry with her natural instincts or worse yet with the mother's parenting?

I was shopping with my infant daughter when a woman working in the store initiated conversation about breastfeeding. "How long do you plan to nurse?" she inquired. Not having given it much thought yet I answered, "I don't know, I guess when her teeth come in, and she's able to chew solid food." Nodding in approval, she offered her opinion, "I've always thought it was very strange when women continue to nurse their babies even when they're older." Glancing down at my daughter I assured the woman that, "Between the two of us I'm sure we'll figure out the timing that is right for us." As I continued to thumb through a clothing rack, a second woman leaned in and said to me, "I nursed my son until he was 29 months, and there is nothing wrong with it!"

A year later, I sat in a café discretely nursing my daughter while chatting with two other mothers. One mother, whose children were grown, commented that her granddaughter had weaned at 12 months and asked when my daughter would be weaning. Just after I'd given my now rehearsed "when she has all of her teeth" answer, the second mother told us that her son had nursed until he was age three. "Three years?!" said the grandmother aghast. "Every mother has to make her own decision," she continued, "but I just think that's unacceptable!"

In a country where only 14% of our babies are breastfed for one full year (as recommended by the American Academy of Pediatrics), breastfeeding toddlers just isn't socially accepted. "Despite the overwhelming positive memories of children who breastfed long enough to remember nursing," comments Jennifer Margulis, Ph.D., a mother of two nurslings (*Mothering* magazine, Nov./Dec. 2002), "American culture has a clear and categorical bias against nursing older children. 'If they're old enough to ask for it, they're too old to be nursing' is the oft-repeated adage. It's as if Americans fear that if a child is cognizant—able to speak and remember—there's something inappropriate even obscene about nursing."

This collective voice of fear-based bias is so often parroted by the people of our lives: friends, family members, physicians, and even strangers. The anti-breastfeeding sentiment around us can be so all-encompassing that it becomes very difficult for us to follow even our own maternal feelings on the issue. I have heard the painful regrets of mothers who felt pressured into weaning their children before they themselves would have otherwise chosen to do so.

In my own experience, I have found the anti-breastfeeding bias to be so subtle at times that it was difficult to detect and therefore to separate from my own voice. Like many breastfeeding women in this country, I entered the nursing relationship thinking in terms of a maximum one-year commitment. I never questioned this assumption until I realized that Quinn would still be getting her teeth at age two. I didn't face my own resistant feeling towards extended nursing until I took into account that America's one-year weaning standard has never been based on what our children's biological requirement for breast milk might even be! Instead this standard has followed the age at which it's believed that most babies can then tolerate the addition of cow milk into their diets. Considering the vast difference between cow milk and human milk (not to mention the differences between calves and human offspring), as well as the problems that pasteurized dairy has now been found to cause within our bodies, I knew that replacing my own milk with the altered milk of another species made very little sense to me.

These insights then raised a pivotal question for me, which has remained unaddressed by mainstream nutrition. What might my daughter's body be calling for, when it comes to the timing of her weaning? Might her continued nursing indicate the following of her biological rhythm—the beat of a drum perhaps very different from our modern-day customs? For me and others with these queries, the research of anthropologists and primatologists offers some interesting possibilities. "Extended nursing is actually the norm among primates," says Margulis (in the prior-mentioned article). "World-renowned primatologist Frans de Waal," she continues, "has observed that tandem nursing is common in bonobos, who nurse their young until they are approximately four years old." Her article then directs us to the work of Katherine A. Dettwyler, adjunct professor of anthropology and nutrition at Texas A&M University, researching both nonhuman primates and the infant nursing practices across a variety of cultures. "Dettwyler writes that nursing a four-year-old, or even a six-year-old is both 'normal and natural for humans' and argues that the 'predictions, based on the non-human primate patterns, range between 2.5 and 7.0 years of age.'"

A third resource Margulis offers is Meredith Small, cultural anthropologist at Cornell University. In her book *Our Babies, Ourselves: How Biology and Culture Shape the Way We Parent*, Small refers to human cultures that practice extended breastfeeding and writes, "In all cases, this hominid blueprint of the way babies were fed for 99 percent of human history indicates breast milk as the primary or sole food until two years of age or so, and nursing commonly continuing for several more years. Analysis of the remains of American Indian bones shows definitive evidence that infants were breastfed exclusively for the first year of life and then gradually weaned when they were five years old."

When we look at this greater picture of humanity's historical roots, our present-day weaning patterns across the globe, and even of our other primate relatives, we see that the current industrialized lifestyle has turned the tables considerably. What we now refer to as "extended" nursing has actually always been the standard, and the modern trend toward early weaning is not in fact the only appropriate way of doing things but is, in all honesty, a cultural anomaly.

This was good news for my daughter and me. I began to realize that the anxiety I was experiencing around the continued nursing of my toddler was due solely to societal pressures. When I saw the larger picture, I was able to unload a fretful bias, to honor my little one's body-wisdom, and to find a resting place in my own maternal intuition. No longer bogged down by worry, I can now simply enjoy the richness of our bond together and trust in her and in myself to indeed work out our very own perfect timing.

✤ FEEDING TODDLERS:
SPECIAL DIETARY CONSIDERATIONS

Just like when they were infants, our little toddlers have unique feeding needs of their own. Unlike when they were doubling their body weight in a matter of weeks, however, food may become less of a priority. Not only has their growth rate slowed down (and therefore their requirements of food) but many toddlers, busy at play, simply don't want to sit still long enough to eat an entire meal.

Your baby may have a bit more to say now about what she thinks is "yummy" or "yucky." At one to two years old she is just beginning to discover her own autonomy, and what enters her mouth is one of the few things over which she has some control. At an age that is said to thrive on having structure, some toddlers may request to eat the same foods everyday, as a way of creating a routine that is comforting to them. Younger palates are more sensitive than ours as well, so it takes a while longer to get used to new tastes and textures.

Seeking to honor our little ones' independent choices while at the same time ensuring their nutritional needs are met can be a bit of a dance. Here are some helpful hints for low-stress toddler feeding:

1. Have food available for snacking throughout the day. This is not only accommodating to toddlers on the go. Two-year-old tummies fill up quickly; they need to eat smaller amounts more frequently in order to get all the nutrition they need.

2. Start out with small portions (one-and-a-half to two tablespoons per food item). Unlike adults who often overestimate the amount of food needed, young children are often a better judge of how much is enough. Offering tiny tastes can make new food less intimidating as well. At seventeen months, our Quinn wouldn't try a new food if it resembled something that she had previously tried and hadn't cared for. If I thought that she might really like it, I'd just dab a little on her lip so she wouldn't miss out on a new yummy flavor. She would probe it with her tongue and usually welcome more.

3. Respect your child's right to preference of food, even if you can't always accommodate it. Not always being able to give your child what he wants is inevitable, but showing disapproval of his personal likes or dislikes can be shaming and can create negative associations around certain foods (foods that he may otherwise decide that he likes at some point in the future). Like big people, little ones are more receptive of trying new things when they feel their own perspective is valued.

4. Continue to offer new foods at family meals, but also have something on the table that you know they will eat. Let her know that she is always welcome to try anything set on the table. One day she may just surprise you! It's important that young children have a positive experience with food and sharing in communal meals.

5. Speak positively about your child's eating habits. What we say about our children they believe (and act out). Children often get labeled as "finicky" or "picky" eaters, but as Lisa Tracy points out in the book *Kid Food*, "You risk programming yourselves and your children for more rejection in this way. . . . View the fussiness as an event rather than as an ongoing problem and things will go better," she advises. "Instead of verbally confirming that your son does not like peas, simply say 'Oh, no peas tonight. Another time.'"

6. Role play together about trying new foods. Switching roles is generally good for a giggle. Pretend that you (or a puppet/doll) are the one that's apprehensive of new foods. Make silly sounds and expressions when a plate is offered to you, then eventually relent and try a nibble. Tastes can be met with an "mmmm...that's good" and others with "no thank you."

7. Spend time together growing and preparing your food! Age two is just old enough to watch sprouts grow or practice stirring together ingredients in a bowl. Whatever garden or kitchen activities you can do together will pique your toddler's interest in new foods.

8. Children are more receptive to trying new things when they aren't feeling any pressure to do so. Sometimes just the feeling of being watched is enough to make a young child shy away from taking that first courageous bite. One mother told me the following story about her little girl who at the time wouldn't eat anything green (not even green colored Jell-O, but she would eat the other colors). The family was at a restaurant together and the mother wanted her daughter to try a new food. "Eeeeeeew," the little girl squealed and wouldn't take one bite. When the mother returned, however, she was met with her daughter's clean plate and a request for more.

9. Continued breastfeeding is an excellent way to help meet our toddler's needs. As a nursing baby grows older, the nutrients of his mother's milk become more highly concentrated. This way baby still receives high nutrition as the frequency of nursing decreases. Those one or two sleepy breastfeedings at nap and bedtime help make up for what may have been missing from the day's food intake. For the toddler who is still getting in teeth and cannot yet fully chew a variety of solids, this is of particular importance.

❧ FAT

Fat is an essential dietary component for babies and toddlers. Breast milk, which is an abundant source of health-promoting fat, naturally meets this need. More and more, it is being recommended that cooked oils (and animal fats) be avoided. Unlike these processed fats, however, which are transformed by high temperatures, the fats of raw foods show no harmful effects on the arteries or the heart!

Here are some raw and fabulous sources of necessary fat: soaked nuts and seeds—these can be blended into milks, pates, dips, whips, smoothies, etc.; nut/seed butters—such as almond, pumpkin seed, macadamia, sunflower, and tahini; fatty "fruits"—avocados and olives (sun-dried/cured olives can be soaked to cut down on the added salt content); and cold-pressed oils—such as olive, hempseed, flaxseed or coconut.

Some families also include the occasional use of organic, raw, goat milk in their living-foods diet. In *Sunfood Success Diet*, David Wolfe suggests this calcium source for the young child who is not yet eating a diet rich in fresh leafy greens.

❧ SNEAKY GREENS

As a toddling baby begins to nurse less and to gain more nutrition from solids, getting a variety of greens in her diet becomes more essential. In a plant-based diet leafy greens are the major source of calcium and iron. Greens also help to maintain healthy blood-sugar levels as well as a proper pH balance within the body. Grown-up salads, however, can be unappealing or difficult for a young toddler to chew. Here are some recipe ideas with which we've had success (see "Recipes for Children" section for the "Kids' Salad").

Banana in a Blanket

Yields 2 servings.

> 2 generous teaspoons almond or pumpkinseed butter
> (or desired amount)
> 2 lettuce leaves
> 1 banana

Spread nut/seed butter onto each of the lettuce leaves. Cut the banana in half and place it in the center of the buttered leaf. Swaddle the banana in the leafy "blanket" and serve. If the lettuce leaves are small, cut the banana into thirds before wrapping.

Variation: Sprinkle in some soaked sunflower seeds.

Grasshopper Smoothie

Yields 1 adult and 1 child-sized serving.

> 1 frozen banana, cut into chunks
> 1 cup fresh pineapple
> ½ cup fresh pineapple juice (or water)
> 1 ounce fresh wheat grass juice
> Sprig of fresh mint

Combine all ingredients together in a blender and blend until smooth (add more juice/water to thin).

Substitution: If fresh organic pineapple is not available, dried pineapple makes a fine substitution. Soak the pineapple overnight and use both the fruit and the soak water.

Apple-Green Juice

Yields 1 adult and 1 child-sized serving.

3 apples
1 medium-sized cucumber
2–3 leaves swiss chard or spinach
Small lemon wedge (peeled)

Juice all ingredients. Stir and serve "as is" or freeze into juicicles.

Papaya with Wheat Grass

½ cup ripe papaya
2 teaspoons fresh wheat grass juice

Cut the fresh papaya length-wise and scoop out the seeds. Discard the seeds or save for use in grown-up salads. (Papaya seeds are radish-like in flavor.) Next, scoop out enough papaya to fill ½ cup. Mash it with a fork then mix in wheat grass juice, or for a smoother blend, puree both ingredients together in a blender adding small amounts of water if necessary.

Variation: Add ½ teaspoon dehydrated barley green.

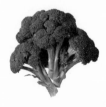

Sprout Pots for Tots

Grow edible houseplants! Sunflower and buckwheat seeds both need soil to grow green sprouts. I like to have decorative pots bulging with green sprouts in sunny spots in the house. Down within a toddler's reach, they can sneak a little whenever they want. (Big floor pots help to avoid over-tipped plants.) My neighbor says that her daughter started eating sprouts because of my tot-pots, and that I *must* include them in this book!

Veggie Wraps/Sandwiches

If bread plays a favored role in your family diet, try packing it full of fresh veggies.

This is our daughter's favorite way to devour a wide variety of leafy greens.

Whole grain tortilla, pita, or sprouted bread, warmed or
toasted
Vegan mayo, hummus, avocado, or dressing of choice

Fresh veggie medley of choice: cucumber, lettuce, baby asparagus spears, kale, swiss chard, spinach, bok choy, beet greens, minced broccoli, broccoli greens, ripe bell pepper strips (red, yellow, or orange), sprouts (alfalfa, mung bean, lentil, sunflower green, or buckwheat lettuce) grated carrot, grated zucchini, or pitted olives.

Top the bread with your dressing of choice and then fill your sandwich or wrap full of different vegetables; the larger the variety of colors, the better.

Banana-Yogurt-Spirulina Pops

As with miso, soy yogurt is not a raw food. However, it does contain living cultures beneficial for digestion. (Nancy's Organic brand has a vegan version that is free of sugar-cane sweeteners.)

2 cups yogurt-style cultured soy
1 banana, mashed
2–4 teaspoons raw agave nectar or sweetener of choice
2 teaspoons spirulina powder (add more if desired)
14 mini-Popsicle sticks (available in craft supplies stores)

In a small to medium-sized bowl, mix all the ingredients together using a spoon or fork. Next, spoon the mixture into an ice-cube tray and insert Popsicle sticks. (A child as young as age two can help to stir, spoon, and stick!) Freeze until solid, and then transfer the pops to a freezer bag for freshness.

Variation: To make a simpler spirulina-swirl pop, omit the banana when mixing together the cultured soy, sweetener, and spirulina. Fold in an additional cup of cultured soy, creating a swirled effect. Stick and freeze.

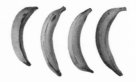

Recipes for Children

Mix a little foolishness with your prudence. It's good to be silly at the right moment.

— Horace

There are self-protective instincts in young children which impel them to seek foods needed at the moment by their body cells. I made a study of children under ten years of age who lived on Vermont farms, in order that I might learn the workings of these instincts. I discovered that these young farm children chewed cornstalks, ate raw potatoes, raw green apples, ripe apples, the grapes that grow wild throughout the state, sorrel, timothy grass heads, and the part of the timothy stem that grows underground. They ate salt from the cattle box, drank water from the . . . trough . . . and, by the handful, a dairy-ration supplement containing seaweed; they even filled their pockets with this, to eat during school. . . . When the children discovered the [apple cider] vinegar they would take a dip of it in the cup and drink it.

If we were wise enough to carry over into adult life the instincts of childhood, we would make a point of eating fruit, berries, edible leaves, and edible roots that would not be cooked.

— D.C. Jarvis, M.D., *Folk Medicine*

Serving as a childcare provider now within my home (Mama Green's Children's Garden), I'm discovering the joy of tickling more little taste buds. Caring for children from diverse dietary lifestyles, I initially thought I was in for quite a challenge. It's been my experience, however, that with few exceptions, children are quite naturally raw-foods enthusiasts! There do seem to be some secrets in providing the right opportunity. Here are a few that I've stumbled upon:

1. *Keep it simple:* Great news, you don't have to be a raw-food gourmet to find your children smacking their lips. In fact, the more complex the recipe the less acceptance it very well may receive.

2. *Mild seasonings:* We might think it bland, but a child's senses are generally more acute than ours. (It is said that we loose a few taste buds as well as some sense of smell as we grow older.) Very strong, pungent, or spicy seasonings are frequently a turn-off (comparable to what we moms may experience during pregnancy). For this reason, I decrease amounts of garlic, onion, ginger, and other strong fresh seasonings when preparing for children. I may also replace them with dried herbs to cut down on the intensity.

3. *Happy associations:* Who honestly really likes something just because we're told it's good for us? Even we grown-ups go for living foods because of all the happy associations: vibrant flavors, increased energy, new experiences of health and healing, new feelings of joy/overall well-being, etc. Children may not always be cognizant of the connection between how their bodies feel and the foods that they eat (or adults for that matter), but they do know what's fun! (Hence the power of food advertisements.) Secret number three? Fun and play, fun and play!

   Here are a few good stories to show you just what I mean: On one occasion, I loaded up a wagon full of kids, handed them all a whole raw carrot and said we were going to feed them to the horses. One child started munching his. The others followed. By the time we got to the horses (15 minutes later), there wasn't much left but stubs. Now I bring more carrots.

Another time, I had three little ones in my living room pretending to be kittens. It had been a while since they'd taken a water break and none of them wanted to stop their sweet play. I served us all water in little bowls, showing them how kittens drink, and with lots of giggles they lapped it all up.

I stood with another mother at our community garden when she turned to me and marveled, "My kids eat all kinds of greens when we're here in the garden that they won't touch at home." The two of us deduced that the garden must be an enchanted place.

4. *Variety of choices:* A wide range of foods to choose from is key to a balanced diet. Offering choices also honors our children's need for autonomy and gives more opportunity to respond to their own bodies' promptings. This doesn't have to mean turning every meal into a smorgasbord, but you may want to have a bowl of fruit accessible, for example, have sprout pots growing at child-level and encourage free-roaming in the garden. ("Eat anything edible you want, and as much as you want of it!") When making shared dishes for mealtime, set aside some of the individual ingredients for the children. This also gives them more options if the texture or seasonings of the particular, soup, salad, or pate is unpleasant for them.

During snack-time with my group of kids, I like to have a few plates of simple food items to choose from (this also helps accommodate differing food interests within the group). I tend to serve raw-foods familiars (like apples, pears, peaches, and bananas) and "transitional" foods (rice cakes or popcorn with sea veggies), alongside the more "exotic" foods (such as pomegranate seeds). Here's a list of potential snack bar items (please note that foods such as hard raw vegetables, popcorn, grapes, whole nuts, and dried fruit are considered to be choking hazards for babies and toddlers): cashews, pecans, macadamia nuts, soaked almonds (my preschoolers enjoy peeling them before eating), pumpkin seeds, and pomegranate seeds; fruit slices such as: apple, pear, peach, plum, mango, papaya, or kiwi; orange or grapefruit rounds (these are extra special served with a cherry in the center); fresh pineapple chunks, cherries, grapes (cut in half for the young ones), and berries; raisins and other dried fruit, soaked or unsoaked (cut up large pieces for younger children and follow with brushing teeth to prevent tooth decay); green sprouts (such as buckwheat, sunflower, or mungbean); raw sweet corn (shucked or cut into thirds); thin-sticks of veggies: carrots, celery, jicama, and broccoli stalks served with dressing for dipping; sugar snap peas or snow peas; sun-dried black olives (soaked, you may also want to pit them); cucumber slices, peeled (served with or without dulse flakes); avocado slices, peeled (served with or without dulse flakes); and nori sheets (you may want to cut them into smaller squares, strips, or shapes).

❧ INTRODUCING SALAD TO CHILDREN

On one blessed day with the kids I hadn't finished preparing their food. Their hungry tummies were restless, so I put a heap of dressed lettuce on each of their plates to buy myself a little more time. Each child ate every bite and asked for more and then more! A well-dressed lettuce salad has lots of kid-appeal, but because it takes longer to feel full on lighter bites, we (and our kids) oftentimes grab for something heavier. I've since started serving salad as a first course on a regular basis—upon the children's request!

Kids' Salad

Organic light green lettuce (such as romaine, green leaf, bibb, or butterhead)*

Dressing of choice (see homemade recipes to follow)

Wash lettuce and drain or have a child help to spin it in a salad-spinner. Hand out leaves to helpers and tear bite-sized pieces of lettuce together. Put it all into a salad bowl and toss with your preferred dressing. Serve alone as an appetizer!

Variation: Some children prefer eating salad they can pick up more easily with their hands. Try cutting an organic head of iceberg lettuce into wedges and serve with a small dipping bowl of dressing.

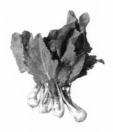

---

*If salad is a new food for your child, I recommend starting with mild-flavored mono-colored leaves. Even red-leaf lettuce can be held suspect by the very cautious connoisseur. Once accepted, gradually introduce bits of darker greens such as spinach, chard, beet, collard, etc. The baby greens tend to be milder than mature greens.

Carrot-Raisin Salad

2 carrots, grated
2 apples, grated
½ lemon, juiced
½ cup raisins, soaked 1–3 hours
½ teaspoon ground cinnamon
⅛ teaspoon ground allspice
⅛ teaspoon ground nutmeg
1 teaspoon fresh ginger juice (optional)
¼ cup chopped pecans or shredded dried coconut
¼ cup fresh or reconstituted dried pineapple chunks (optional)

Toss all ingredients together in a large bowl and serve.

Sweet Angel-Hair Red Beets

This recipe is inspired by a lovely beet salad I once ordered at Ecopo-
lotan, a raw foods restaurant in Minneapolis. If your child opposes
mint leaves or nuts, omit them from his serving.

1 large beet, cut into angel-hair strands with Saladecco-Spiralizer
1–2 tablespoon flaxseed oil, walnut oil (or other cold-pressed oil)
1 tablespoon balsamic vinegar
    (fresh lemon juice or orange juice can substitute)
¼ cup walnut pieces
5 medjool dates, pitted and cut lengthwise into strips
1 small apple, chopped or sliced
Handful of fresh mint, finely minced
1 tablespoon golden flaxseeds

In a medium-sized mixing bowl, toss the angel-hair beet strands with
the oil and balsamic vinegar. Add the walnut pieces and dates and toss
again. Garnish with the apple, mint, and sprinkle of flax seeds.

❧ HOMEMADE DRESSINGS/DIPPING SAUCES

The dressing can make or break the kid-salad. Bottled dressings can be helpful when getting started on raw foods. If you use them, you'll want to make sure to check labels for unwanted ingredients such as sugar, preservatives, and hydrogenated oils. Vegan sugar-free options can be found at natural food stores. (My day-care kids enjoy Annie's Goddess, for example, as well as any of Drew's dairy-free selections.) For endless variety and fresher ingredients definitely play with making your own! The next two sweet dressing recipes come from St. Martin's Table (with slight modification), a vegetarian café in Minneapolis, where they make all of their own salad dressings. (If you ever get the chance to lunch there, be sure to leave a generous tip—each server is a volunteer who hands the gratuity over to organizations aiding world-hunger.)

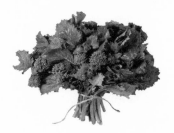

Poppy Seed Dressing

3 tablespoons onion, minced
1 cup raw honey or agave nectar
2 teaspoons sea salt/Celtic salt
¾ cup raw, apple-cider vinegar
1 teaspoon lemon zest
2 teaspoons dry mustard
1 tablespoons fresh lemon juice
2 cups cold-pressed olive oil
3 tablespoons poppy seeds

Blender method: Place all ingredients except the poppy seeds in a blender and blend until smooth (add small amounts of water to thin if necessary). Pour into a large glass jar, add poppy seeds, and shake to mix.

With a food processor: First, mince the onion in the food processor. Next, combine all ingredients except the oil. Process for 3 minutes. Add the oil and process again for 1 minute.

Apple Vinaigrette

¾ cup fresh apple juice
½ cup cold-pressed oil (olive or flax seed)
¼ teaspoon celery seed
¾ cup raw, apple-cider vinegar
½ teaspoon sea salt/Celtic salt
2 teaspoons black pepper (optional—reduce or omit for kids)

No fuss method: In a small mixing bowl (or canning jar) whisk all the ingredients together with small whisk or fork. Cover and refrigerate until serving.

Almond Butter Dipping Sauce

⅓ cup raw almond butter

4 tablespoons Bragg's or Noma Shoyu (raw soy sauce)

½ cup cold-pressed olive oil

2 tablespoons fresh lime juice

¼-inch gingerroot, minced

½ small clove garlic, minced (or ½ teaspoon dried, granulated
   garlic)

Up to ½ cup of purified water

2 tablespoons cilantro, finely minced (optional)

Put all ingredients in a blender and blend until smooth, adding water 1 tablespoon at a time to thin to desired consistency. Add cilantro and pulse to mix.

Variation: Put a teaspoon of cayenne pepper in a batch for the grown-ups.

Ginger-Honey Mustard Dressing

⅓ cup prepared mustard

⅓ cup raw honey

½ cup cold pressed olive or flaxseed oil

Juice of half a lemon

½–1 tablespoon freshly grated gingerroot

¼ cup purified water

Whisk all ingredients together in a small mixing bowl or blend together in a blender.

Mama Green's Tahini Dressing

½ cup raw tahini
½ lemon, juiced
⅓ cup raw, apple-cider vinegar
½ cup sesame oil or olive oil
¼ cup Bragg's or Nama Shoyu
1 teaspoon onion powder
1 teaspoon garlic powder
2 tablespoons parsley, chives, cilantro, or other fresh herbs of
    choice

Whisk all ingredients together in a small mixing bowl or blend together
in a blender.

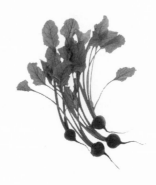

RAWmen Noodle Soup

My instant soup fans really enjoy this recipe. The bouillon cubes match the familiar flavors of the broth base—without the MSG. For a yeast-free, living bouillon try using a mild, fresh miso. For first-time introduction, I recommend this very simple version. More ingredients can be added later on. Participating in the noodle spinning (and the zucchini growing) is a big part of this quick-soup's charm, as well as the comfort of having it served warm.

    2 small zucchini, cut into thirds
        or 2 cups green cabbage, cut into thin strips
    2 cups hot water
    2 cubes vegetable bouillon (by Rapunzel Organics
        or preferred vegetarian bouillon) or one cube
        plus 2 tablespoons Braggs Aminos

Cut the zucchini thirds into angel-hair strands with a Saladecco Spiral-izer or substitute with cabbage strips. Set aside. Heat water and pour into a large ceramic bowl. Crumble the bouillon cubes into the hot water and stir until dissolved. Allow this broth to cool to a comfort-able eating temperature, add zucchini or cabbage "noodles," and serve immediately.

Variation: Add ⅓ cup grated carrot, broccoli stalk, or broccoli florets, 2 teaspoons dulse flakes, and/or baked tofu cubed.

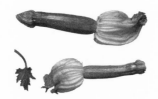

Shish Kebabs

As you've probably determined during State Fair season, just about anything can be eaten off a stick! (If you're tired of the fried-food blues, stick to your family picnic basket this year.) Little ones who are still developing finer motor skills seem to especially appreciate this break from the usual utensils.

Potential ingredients:

> Avocado, cubed (with a light coat of fresh lemon juice, if they
> won't be eaten right away)
> Cherry tomatoes or sliced tomato wedges
> Organic iceberg lettuce cut into small wedges
> Cured black olives, soaked and pitted
> Cucumber slices (peeled)
> Sugar snap peas/snow peas
> Thin carrot slices
> Baked tofu cubes*

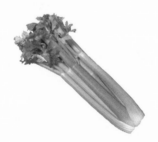

---

*Baked tofu can be found in the refrigerated section at natural foods stores (or in the "natural foods" section of larger grocery stores). This cooked food can be very satisfying for children who are accustomed to eating meat with meals. (One of my pre-schoolers calls it "chicken.")

Also needed:

> A bamboo skewer or chopstick for each person
> Sauce/dressing of choice

Bamboo skewers are thinner and easier to slide food onto. I use chopsticks for younger children, however, to give them more control over the stick and to help avoid getting poked. I've found that with chopsticks it's easiest to place the slice of carrot or cucumber on a cutting board, push the stick down into the center of the round, and gently twist the veggie up onto the stick. Choose from the foods above, add any others you wish, and skewer them alternately until each stick is stacked. Serve with dipping bowls of dressing or drizzle lightly just before serving.

Ants on a Log

You've likely seen this kid-favorite before. Use unroasted nut butter and you've got a quick and satisfying raw snack. Little hands enjoy helping to spread the butter and dot the logs with raisins.

> Celery sticks
> Nut butter*
> Raisins, dried currants, or dried cranberries

Cut the celery sticks to desired length. (The full stalk can be fun for older kids.) Fill the celery stalks with nut butter and spread with a table knife or the rounded back of a spoon. Garnish with a row of raisins.

---

*Almond and pumpkinseed butters can be purchased raw (See Nature's First Law in the "References, Further Reading, and Resources" section). "Raw" cashew butter has technically been heated, but is a tasty alternative to roasted peanut butter.

Lettuce Boats

Any lettuce leaf can be used for making sandwich wraps, but romaine hearts are the best shape for making "boats." Younger children seem to also prefer the crunchy ribbed center of this variety (which is said to have calming properties). Clean, drain (or spin-dry) the lettuce leaves and load with the sandwich filling of your choice. Here are some ideas:

Avocado (plain or with dressing)

Avocado, cured black olives, minced celery, chopped tomato

Hummus or avocado with match-sticked veggies (carrot, celery, bell pepper, etc.) topped with sprouts and drizzled with a dressing of choice

"Save the Tuna Salad" (see "Guest Chef Recipes")
—with or without sprouts

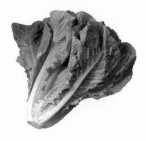

Apple Sandwiches

For a fresh new sandwich idea use sliced apples as you would bread. Select a crisp, juicy variety of apple (Fuji, Braeburn, Spartan, Pink Lady, and Gala are often very good). Avoid anything mushy and mealy. Cut the apples into rounds, then spread and stack with a favored sandwich filling. Here are some ideas:

Raw nut butter, for added nutrition mix in ½ teaspoon fresh-ground flaxseed

Cashew butter, minced celery, raisins

Tahini, honey, sunflower seeds

Almond butter, raisins, lettuce

Almond butter, dried cranberries on a Bosc pear (instead of an apple)

Pumpkinseed butter, sliced banana

"Save the Tuna Salad" (see "Guest Chef Recipes") —lettuce and/or sprouts

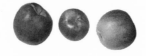

Spiced Pear Rings

Like spiced apples in the jar? Here's a raw version with natural coloring. Apples can be used; however, pear is a much better match in texture.

1 teaspoon whole cloves
1 cinnamon stick
4 bags hibiscus spice tea (I like Yogi Organic teas)
1–2 tablespoons agave nectar (or sweetener of choice)
Purified water
2 fairly firm, yet sweet-to-the-taste pears, cored, sliced into
    rounds, and lightly coated with fresh lemon juice

Place cloves, cinnamon stick, tea bags, and sweetener in a large wide-mouthed canning jar. Fill ⅓ of the jar with water and stir until sweetener is dissolved (if using a granular sweetener). Add the pear rounds and enough additional water to top off the jar. Seal the jar with its lid and leave to marinate in the refrigerator for up to 48 hours.

Zucchini-Applesauce/Fruit Leather

This recipe is especially handy for parents of the solid-food beginner with an older sibling. When making the sauce for baby, omit the cinnamon and extra sweetener. Taste it, then add sweetener and spice for you and older children, if desired. Enjoy as an applesauce or spread the sauce onto Teflex sheets, in a thin layer, and dehydrate until fruit can be easily peeled from the sheets (between 105°–110°F, for 4–6 hours).

    4 apples, cored and peeled
    1 small to medium-sized zucchini, peeled and seeded
    ½ teaspoon ground cinnamon
    2 tablespoons agave syrup (or alternative sweetener)

Making the sauce: If you have a heavy-duty juicer (such as a Champion) this will work the best for achieving an even consistency. Using the blank screen, homogenize the apples and zucchini alternately. Then mix the cinnamon and agave in by hand. If you do not have a homogenizing juicer, process all of the ingredients in a food processor or blender until smooth. (If using a blender, you may have to add small amounts of liquid, such as fruit-juice, to run the blender blades.)

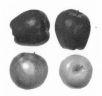

Creamy Strawberry Pudding

This whips up into a rich yogurt-like treat. Mix in extra chopped berries if you like. Yields 2 servings.

1 ½ cup fresh strawberries (or frozen, thawed)
1 cup avocado
½ cup dates, pitted and soaked in ½ cup water 6–8 hours
    (save soak water for recipe)

Blend all ingredients together in a blender adding extra water, date-soak water, or nut milk to thin.

Mud Pies

Yields 4 servings.

¼ cup pecans
2 tablespoons flax seed
1 tablespoon maple syrup
2 avocados
1½ cup dates, pitted and soaked 6–8 hours (in just enough
    water to cover, save soak water for recipe)
2 tablespoons organic cocoa powder (raw carob powder can
    substitute)
4 cherries (optional)

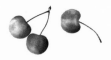

To make a crumb-crust, grind the pecans and flaxseeds into a fine meal. This can be done by pulsing them in a blender or by grinding small batches in an electric coffee grinder. Transfer the ground meal into a mixing bowl and toss together with the maple syrup. This is your crumb-crust. Divide this sweetened ground mixture into 4 dessert cups and set aside. Now put the remaining ingredients into a blender and blend until you have achieved a smooth pudding-like texture (add small amounts of additional date-soak water, maple syrup, nut milk, or water to thin, if needed). Pour the chocolate pudding mixture over the ground pecan mixture in each of the dessert cups. Top with a cherry, if you've got some, and chill until serving.

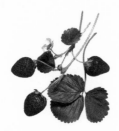

No-Bake Granola Bars

This nutty grain-sprout recipe is a big hit around our kid table. It is however, an exception to the keep-things-simple tip. In order to make this recipe most practical, I recommend sprouting, drying, and storing the dehydrated ingredients ahead of time. This way you don't have to do it all in four consecutive days. You may also want to prepare extra dried ingredients to keep on hand for other recipes—or for your next batch of bars.

Dry ingredients:

> 1 cup wheat berries, spelt, or rye
> 1 cup buckwheat groats
> 1 cup almonds, soaked
> 1 cup dried, shredded coconut
> ½ teaspoon cinnamon
> ¼ teaspoon sea salt
> > (omit if using salted pumpkin-seed butter)
> 1 cup dried apples, chopped
> > (approximately two fresh apples if drying your own)
> 1 cup raisins, chopped or dried currants

Wet ingredients:

> ⅓ cup nut butter*
> ⅓ cup raw honey (no substitutes, as it helps the bar to firm
> > when chilled)
> 5 tablespoons quality coconut oil
> 1 teaspoon vanilla (optional)

---

*If your kids are used to the taste of peanut butter, you may want to use it for introducing this recipe. You'll want to make sure that your brand does not contain sugar or hydrogenated oils.

Day 1: Soak the buckwheat groats.

Day 2: Drain and rinse the buckwheat groats. Store in a sprouting jar or colander and rinse at least twice daily. Start the wheat (or preferred grain berry) and almonds soaking separately.

Day 3: Drain and rinse the wheat berries and almonds. Store the soaked wheat berries in a sprouting jar or colander (and rinse twice daily). Chop the almonds finely. Next, dehydrate the chopped almonds along with the buckwheat sprouts at 110°F for 4 hours or until crunchy. If drying your own apples, chop and dehydrate these also. They require about the same drying time.

Day 4: Place the jar of coconut oil in a small bowl of warm water to start liquefying the oil. (The entire jar need not liquefy, only enough for the recipe.) Set aside. In a large mixing bowl combine all of the dry ingredients (see list above) together and stir to mix thoroughly. Set aside. In a medium-sized bowl, measure and pour the liquified coconut oil. Now add the remaining wet ingredients to the oil and whisk together with a fork. Next, pour the wet ingredient mixture into the dry ingredients using a spatula to scrape the sides of the bowl. Mix thoroughly and pour into an 8-inch x 8-inch glass cake pan (a glass pie plate will also work fine). Press the granola bar mixture down firmly and chill in the refrigerator or freezer until solid. Cut into bars and serve.

Variations: Substitute some or all of the grain berries with sunflower seeds, sesame seeds, or rolled oats. Also try using other favorite dried fruits in place of the apple and raisins.

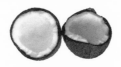

Painted Easter Candies

This one is inspired by the recipe "Touchstone Caramels" found in the raw dessert book *Sweet Temptations* by Frances Kendall. Here I make these buttery sweets into miniature Easter eggs. They can also be formed into cubes or balls for other times of year. (For winter holiday, they make nice white "snow balls.") If your kitchen helpers are very young, make the juice coloring ahead of time as well as shaping the egglets. They'll enjoy helping to dye the coconut and then choosing which colors to roll the candies through.

¾ cup pine nuts (raw cashews can substitute)
2 cups dates, softened slightly by pre-soaking 3–5 hours,
     drained and pitted
2 teaspoons pure vanilla extract
2 cups dried shredded coconut

Fresh juice options for coloring:

Lavender/blue—blueberries*
Pink—raspberry*
Hot pink—red beet
Yellow—carrot or yellow beet
Green—wheat grass or parsley

---

*Berry juice can be easily extracted by pressing the berries into a fine mesh sieve with the round back of a spoon. If using fresh-frozen berries, simply thaw and collect the juice.

Put the pine nuts, dates, and vanilla in a food processor and process using the s-blade until smooth. (You may need to add a small amount of the date-soak water to achieve a smooth consistency.) Transfer into a large mixing bowl and mix in half of the shredded coconut (1 cup) with a spoon. Chill for one hour to firm and form into ½ teaspoon-sized eggs or desired shape. (For eggs, I roll them into balls first and then gently pinch one end.) Set out a saucer or small bowl for each color and divide the remaining cup of shredded coconut amongst them. Add just a few drops of each coloring juice and stir. Now roll candies into the tinted coconut. (Mix leftover colored coconut together, and you've got pretty confetti sprinkles! Store refrigerated in an airtight container and use for topping banana ice cream or other desserts.)

Easter basket ideas: Save your berry baskets (you know those little plastic green ones). School-age children can weave them with ribbons and/or dress them up with fresh flowers. Manufactured bird's nest baskets (available in craft supply stores) are also charming. I like to skip the plastic grass altogether and use real wheat grass and/or edible flowers and berries.

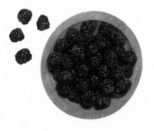

❧ Frozen Treats

Raspberry Yogurt Mini-Pops

2 cups cultured soy yogurt (Nancy's Organic brand is
   recommended)
1–2 tablespoon agave nectar (or sweetener of choice)
¾ cup fresh raspberries (or frozen, thawed)
   mashed with a fork
12–14 mini-Popsicle sticks

Stir all food ingredients together. Next, spoon the raspberry yogurt mixture into an ice-cube tray and insert sticks. Freeze until solid then transfer to a freezer bag. Return to the freezer until serving.

Tray options: I find that these 1-ounce ice-cube-tray servings are just the right size for toddlers and preschoolers (they're generally able to eat it all before it drips all over their hands). For older children, there are some great Popsicle trays on the market for making homemade Popsicles. Double this recipe if you're using a larger tray.

Neapolitan Ice Cream—Thank you Delphine Rigault-Noel!

Vanilla

2 cups fresh, young coconut pulp
1 cup fresh, young coconut water
2 tablespoons coconut butter
3 or 4 tablespoons vanilla extract
¼ cup agave nectar (optional)

Chocolate

   2 cups fresh, young coconut pulp
   1 cup fresh, young coconut water
   2 tablespoons coconut butter
   ½–¾ cup tightly packed, peeled, and ground cacao beans
   ½-¾ cup agave nectar

Strawberry

   2 cups liquefied strawberries
   1 cup fresh, young coconut pulp
   2–4 tablespoons coconut butter
   ¼–½ cup agave nectar

Blend each batch separately, and put into 1 gallon-size Ziploc bags or pour into small-sized ice-cube trays (that will fit into a Champion juicer) and freeze overnight. Process through the Champion separately, rinsing the juicer between each flavor, and ideally, re-freeze immediately for 1 to 3 hours. Do not over freeze or the ice cream will become rock hard again. Serve one scoop of each with fresh strawberries.

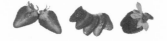

Peppermint Ice Cream by Delphine Rigault-Noel

2 cups fresh, young coconut pulp
1 cup fresh, young coconut water
¼ or more cup agave nectar
Approximately 20 drops peppermint essential oil
½ or more teaspoons vanilla extract

Blend all ingredients together in a BlendTec, freeze at least overnight, process through a Champion juicer with the blank plate, and, ideally, refreeze for another 1–3 hours. Enjoy!

Banana Ice Cream

Yields 3–4 servings.

6 ripe bananas

Peel bananas before freezing in freezer bags. In a heavy-duty juicer, using the blank screen, homogenize the frozen bananas, catching the ice cream in a chilled bowl. It's best eaten right-away but can be stored for a short time in a sealed container in the freezer and then set out to soften for a few minutes before serving. If you don't have a homogenizing juicer, you can use a food processor for a thinner version.

Variation: Add some frozen berries or sliced peaches (running them alternately with the banana through the juicer).

Banana Pops

Banana ice cream just got easier: Cut bananas in half, stick them with Popsicle sticks (standard size), then freeze inside freezer bags.

Watermelon Snow Cones

I absolutely love this recipe! You end up with pink-red snow, and even better than the sugar-syrup version of my childhood, every bite is flavorful. (And by the way, this is also a fabulous way to make use of those sweet but softer-textured melons. They freeze-up just great.)

Sole ingredient: 4 cups sweet, ripe watermelon,
cut into chunks and seeds removed

Put the watermelon chunks in a blender and pulse to liquefy. Pour the watermelon liquid into a glass or ceramic pie plate or a non-aluminum baking dish. Place the dish in the freezer. Return to the dish every 30–45 minutes to stir and mash the ice with a fork as it freezes. This creates small air pockets that will result in a fine crystalline texture (snow). When the mixture starts to freeze around the edges, break this up with the fork. Repeat this periodically until the ice is firm (3–5 hours). Serve watermelon ice in a bowl with spoon or scooped into paper cones.

Variation: To make a watermelon slushee, pour your strained watermelon liquid into ice-cube trays rather than a shallow dish. To make this melting-snow-like drink you need not stir the ice as it's freezing. Simply allow the liquid to freeze just until cubes have partially hardened. Now transfer the watermelon ice-cubes back into the blender and pulse until "slushified."

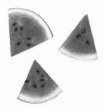

Mixed-Fruit Party Cubes

Before pouring the water to make ice-cubes, place a piece of fresh fruit in each section of the tray. The end result is a medley of dazzling ice-cubes, each with a treat inside! Display them in a serving bowl or in the drinking glasses themselves. Serve with fresh-squeezed lemonade, sun tea, or a homemade fruit juice-seltzer water punch.

Here are some good fruits to choose from:

- *Kiwi fruit—sliced and quartered*
- *Strawberries—halved*
- *Blueberries, raspberries, mulberries, or blackberries*
- *Grapes—halved*
- *Mango, peach, apricot, or pineapple—cut into chunks*
- *Melon (any variety)—scooped into balls or cut into chunks*

Variation: In place of or mixed in with these fruit cubes, make pretty party-ice with fresh mint leaves and/or edible flowers (unsprayed mild varieties such as pansies or rose petals).

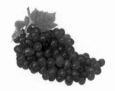

❦ KIDDIE COCKTAILS/BEVERAGES

Creamy Melon-Seed Drink

1 small to medium-sized sweet green melon such as casaba or
    honeydew
Juice of one lime (optional)
1 teaspoon zest of lime (optional)
1 thin sliver fresh gingerroot (optional)
    or 1–2 springs fresh mint

Cut the melon in half, scoop out all the seeds, and put them into the
blender. Add half of the melon flesh, lime juice, zest, and ginger and
blend to liquefy. Strain out the pulp through a nut-milk bag or other
very fine strainer. Discard the pulp. Serve this beverage over crushed
or cubed ice.

Variations: To make a creamy melon soup, simply add the remaining
melon flesh and blend until smooth. Garnish with fresh mint leaves.
Also try using cantaloupe with a dash of cinnamon in place of the
ginger/mint.

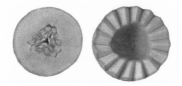

Nut/Seed Milks

1 cup soaked (8–12 hours) raw almonds, sunflower seeds, sesame seeds, walnuts, pecans, or any combination of these

    3 cups purified water (add more for a thinner milk)
    2–3 dates
    1 tablespoon raw honey or alternative sweetener (optional)
    Pinch sea salt/Celtic salt (optional)

Blend all ingredients together in a blender until thoroughly liquified. Strain through a fine sieve or nut-milk bag to remove the pulp. (Fresh pulp can be stored for same-day recipes or dehydrated for further use.) Store refrigerated in a sealed container (keeps for up to two days). Separation of nut/seed milk occurs naturally. Shake or stir to re-mix. Use as you would cow milk or other dairy substitutes. (Nut milks also make a nice foamy froth when blending. I use this for topping Chai tea with almond milk.)

Variation: For added nutrition and flavor, add 2 tablespoons whole flaxseeds (golden or brown) to your nut/seed milks before blending.

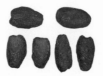

Licuados

A licuado is a simple Mexican-style shake. It is traditionally made by blending cow's milk and sugar with fresh or frozen fruit, nuts, or cocoa powder. A touch of vanilla and a few ice-cubes are also often tossed into the mix. Raw nut/seed milks make delicious licuados. I recommend starting with 2 cups of almond, sunflower, or pecan milk, adding 2–3 dates (or other sweetener), 1 teaspoon vanilla, and any of the following ingredient options:

- *For a licuado de fresa:* add 1 cup fresh or frozen strawberries

- *Un licuado de coco:* ¼–½ cup fresh or dried, shredded coconut meat

- *Un licuado de platano:* one fresh or frozen banana

- *Un licuado de chocolate:* 2 tablespoons organic cocoa powder (raw carob powder can substitute)

Variations: Combine any of the above ingredients and/or any other favorite flavors.

❧ Fresh Fruit and Vegetable Juices

Juice bars are now appearing in shopping malls and natural food stores here in North America, but fresh fruit and veggie juices are also commonly served as a traditional beverage in parts of Mexico. (As I walked in downtown Mexico City for example, I was greeted by little juice bar stands everywhere.) If you've never been to a juice bar, you've got to try it! Ask what's popular and start with something mild (especially for kids). Here are a few fresh recipes for your fruit and veggie juice extractor at home. Juice according to the manufacturer's instructions of your juicer.

Fresh-Squeezed O.J. with Wheat Grass

Wheat grass juice has a naturally sweet and very potent flavor. Many adults consume it straight for its jolt of nutrient-rich, energy-boosting properties. The kids and I like to take it nice and easy in combination with fruit juice. (See also the recipe for "Grasshopper Smoothie" in the "Toddler Foods" section.)

2–3 ounces fresh wheat grass juice
5–6 oranges

If you have a manual wheat-grass juicer this recipe is fun to make with children. Grow a patch of wheat grass (or another cereal green such as barley, spelt, or oat grass) in your garden or windowsill or purchase a flat from a natural food store. Preschoolers can help to cut the grass with small rounded kid-scissors and even younger children can practice putting clippings into the hopper and turning the crank. After you've halved the oranges, little hands can do the squeezing on a manual citrus juicer. Stir the two juices together. This is best served with a child-sized pitcher (measuring pitchers work well) and small juice glasses.

Parsley Lemon-Limeade

One bunch parsley
½ lemon, peeled
1 small lime (or ½ large lime), peeled
5 apples, quartered and seeds removed

Juice, stir, and serve.

All-Orange Smoothie

1 cup fresh carrot juice
1 cup fresh orange juice
1 cup frozen papaya chunks
1 cup frozen mango chucks

Combine all ingredients in a blender and puree until "smooth-ie."

Variation: Replace mango or papaya with fresh pineapple pieces or simply add them.

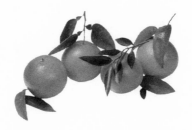

Raspberry Ginger Ale

This makes a special soda treat and aids an upset tummy. Yields 2 large servings.

 1 lemon wedge, peeled
 ¼-½-inch slice fresh gingerroot
 ½ cup fresh raspberries
 ½ cup frozen raspberries

Any of the following sweet fruits:

3 apples, 3 cups grapes, 3 cups fresh pineapple
 Sparkling water

Juice the sweet fruit of choice, lemon, ginger, and the ½ cup fresh raspberries. Divide the juice among the glasses and top off with sparking water. Toss a few frozen raspberries into each glass and serve.

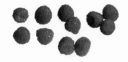

❧ GUEST CHEF: CHAD SARNO

Chad Sarno, certified chef, instructor, and founder of Vital Creations LLC Chef Services has been very active within the raw, vegan community for many years. Most recently Sarno has been executive chef at the Tree of Life Rejuvenation Center and staff chef at the Living Light Culinary Arts Institute. Sarno has been traveling the globe assisting in the ground work of kitchen layout, menu development, and chef training for some of the top restaurants and resorts that specialize in fine living-foods cuisine such as: Roxanne's Restaurant, world's first fine-dining raw-foods restaurant in Larkspur, CA; The Farm Resort and Spa, one of the top five-star spas in Asia; Vitalities Inc., exclusive resort and spa in Kauai, HI; Botanica Restaurant, an organic, raw-foods experience; Tree of Life Rejuvenation Center, Dr. Gabriel Cousen's facility in Patagonia, AZ.

Sarno is developing a reference book, *The Raw Chef: A Journey Through the Senses.* Packed into over 250 pages are some of the most informative charts and quick reference guides to recipe development. From simple secrets to complex techniques—this book will be a superb teaching tool for all skill levels in raw-and-living culinary artistry. It contains detailed herb and spice references, along with a step-by-step process on the simplicity of gourmet spice and flavor combining, and over 225 first- to fifth-course recipes. Thanks to Chad for sharing some of his favorite recipes for kids!

❧ GUEST CHEF RECIPES

All recipes copyright © Vital Creations, LLC (published in Chad Sarno's workbook, *Vital Creations: An Organic Life Experience*).

Macadamia Porridge with Tahitian Vanilla Bean

Yields 3–4 servings.

    2 cups macadamia nuts
    1 cup coconut meat
    3 cups coconut water
    2 apples, 1 chopped, 1 diced
    1 teaspoon Tahitian vanilla bean
    ½ teaspoon Celtic sea salt

Put all the ingredients, except the diced apple, into a high-speed blender and blend until smooth. Mix in the diced apple, by hand. Serve with chopped or blended fruit.

Variations: Substitute any soaked nuts for the macadamias. Also, if coconuts are not available, simply omit them.

Seed Granola

Yields 4 cups.

    1 cup pecans, soaked 10–12 hours
    1 cup almonds, soaked 10–12 hours
    1 cup pumpkin seeds, soaked 10–12 hours
    1 cup sunflower seeds, soaked 10–12 hours
    3 cups sweetener paste (date, raisin, or prune)
    2 apples, diced small
    2 tablespoon cinnamon, ground
    1 teaspoon Celtic sea salt

When all the nuts are soaked, strain off excess water. Using the food processor, pulse all nuts until coarsely ground. Set aside. Also, using the food processor, blend the sweetener with a small amount of water until it becomes a smooth paste. Toss the paste along with the diced apples, cinnamon, and salt with the nut mixture. Hand mix well. Continue by spreading the "wet" granola onto dehydrator sheets and dehydrate at 105°F for 10–12 hours.

Serve with nut milk. Seed granola will keep for months in a sealed container.

Mesquite Nut Milk

Yields 2 servings.

1 cup nut of choice, soaked 10–12 hours
½ cup coconut meat
3 cups coconut water
2 tablespoons mesquite powder
1 teaspoon cinnamon

In blender, blend all ingredients well for 25–20 seconds. Continue by pouring the mixture into a nut-milk bag and squeezing out milk. Chill and serve.

Save the Tuna Salad

Yields 4 servings.

1 cup almonds, soaked 10–12 hours
1 cup sunflower seeds, soaked 10–12 hours
1½ tablespoon dill, fresh and minced
1 tablespoon oregano, fresh and minced
1 teaspoon sage, fresh and minced
2 tablespoons lemon juice
1 tablespoon kelp granules
½ teaspoon Celtic salt
1 teaspoon black pepper
⅓ cup celery minced
¼ cup red onion minced
⅓ cup pickles diced

Homogenize almonds and sunflower seeds. Hand mix in remaining ingredients, mixing thoroughly. Serve by itself or wrapped in nori with assorted veggies.

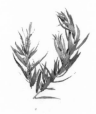

Apple Cake

Yields 6 servings.

2 cups apple, fresh and shredded
1½ cups dried apple, minced
1½ cups pecans, soaked, dehydrated, and ground into flour
¼ cup raisins
1 cup raisins, soaked 2–4 hours and blended into a paste or
    dates pitted
1½ tablespoons cinnamon
2 tablespoons mesquite powder
Nutmeg to taste
¼ teaspoon Celtic salt

Place all the ingredients into a mixing bowl and hand mix gently, yet
thoroughly; set aside. Using a 6-inch spring-form pan, line the bottom with plastic wrap. Press "cake" into pan firmly. Frost with coconut
crème. Chill before serving. Note, with extra cake, form into bars and
dehydrate for 10–12 hours for a great snack on the trail.

Coconut Crème

1 cup coconut meat
½ cup coconut water
½ cup cashews, soaked 10–12 hours
⅓ cup dates, pitted
1 teaspoon vanilla bean
½ teaspoon Celtic salt

In high-speed blender, blend all ingredients until smooth.

Serve as frosting for apple spice cake.

Family Activities

Short and simple makes for a more lasting impression. Children's minds really don't need a lot of words and explanations. Adult minds do!

— Peggy J. Jenkins, P.H.D., *Nurturing Spirituality in Children*

I hear—I forget
I see—I remember
I do—I understand

— Chinese proverb

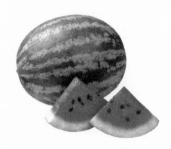

❧ FUN AND GAMES

Bunny Rabbit Buffet

This one's for the little ones.

Supplies needed:

- ❧ Storybook that features a rabbit in a garden (such as *The Tales of Peter Rabbit*)

- ❧ Cotton balls

- ❧ Masking tape

- ❧ Small plates or bowls containing various rabbit foods such as: lettuce, snap peas, carrots, radishes, baby greens, parsley, strawberries, etc. (you may want to choose foods that are listed in your storybook)

- ❧ Use little loops of tape to stick on cottontails for the kids. Hop over to a set table or picnic blanket where your little bunnies can nibble along with the story.

Watermelon Seed-Spitting Challenge

Supplies needed:

- ❧ Watermelon wedges with seeds

- ❧ Small cups

Here's a fun summer party game. Pass out the fresh watermelon wedges and cups for saving the seeds. For a cooperative rather than competitive activity, encourage sharing techniques as a group in order for everyone to beat his/her own record. (I would discourage taking down measurements and keeping score.) Challenge your spitters to top the world record: 66 feet, 11 inches—farther than the length of a bowling alley with one spit!!

❧ BANQUET FOR THE SENSES

This sensory awareness game appears in the book *Ultimate Kid* by Jeffrey Goelitz. The use of blindfolds helps to provide a clear perception of each item the children will experience without the influence of preconceived ideas of how they may taste, feel, sound, or smell (similar to what it's like to be a baby on a sensory level). While evoking feelings of excitement and anticipation, this activity helps to deepen sensitivity to each of the senses. This connects children with their more instinctual nature, paving the way for increased receptivity of their bodies' messages. These skills will serve children well as they grow older and begin to make more food selection choices for themselves.

Preparation:

1. Blindfolds for everyone

2. Dishes, plates, paper cups to hold different objects and foods

3. At least four different sources of smell: spices, herbs, flowers, essential oils, vanilla, other foods, etc.

4. Four sources of touch: a rough rock, smooth stone, waxy leaf, piece of cotton, sponge, sandpaper, velvet, etc.

5. Four sources of taste: various pieces of fruit (both sweet and sour), cinnamon, honey, carob, salt, etc.

6. Four sources of sound: bell, woodblocks, sandpaper, whistle, gong, trickle of water poured from one bowl to another, etc.)

7. Napkins

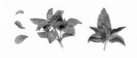

Procedure:

1. Hand out napkins to all children.

2. Have everyone blindfolded and request quiet in the room.

3. Begin by creating the different sources of sound, one by one.

4. Pass around the various objects of smell.

5. Next, pass around, one at a time, the different objects collected for the sense of touch.

6. Pass around the plate that contains different items of taste, encouraging the children to use napkins if their hands get sticky.

7. Request that the children take off their blindfolds and be aware of the first thing that catches their visible attention.

Taste-Bud Trick

Here's a fun guessing game that also tunes into the senses. (Thanks to the June 2002 issue of *Family Fun* magazine for this idea and science experiment #3).

Objects needed:

🍂 Paper-thin slices of raw white potato, apple, and pear

Have your child close her eyes and hold her nose while you give her a sample of each thinly sliced food. Without the sense of smell (or sight) to prompt the taste buds, you may have some surprising results!

🌱 Kitchen Crafts

Fruit and Veggie Stamping

The artwork found in the middle of fresh fruits and vegetables makes great natural stamps for frameable prints, homemade greeting cards, or wrapping paper. By using acrylic or fabric paints you can also decorate cloth napkins, tablecloths, t-shirts, and other fabrics.

Materials:

Assortment of fresh fruit and vegetables: bell pepper, cucumber slices, crook neck squash, broccoli, onions, citrus fruits, artichokes, mushrooms, and walnut shells are all good options

- 🌱 Tempera paint (or acrylic/fabric paint)
- 🌱 Plate or tray to hold the paint
- 🌱 Paper
- 🌱 Newspaper or oilcloth

Prepare your work surface area with newspaper or oilcloth. Cut your fruits and veggies into halves. Pour a moderate amount of paint onto plates or trays. Next, dip your "stamps" into the paint and press them in place onto the paper. To avoid mixing the colors together, allow one color to dry before adding another tint of paint.

Further ideas: Adults and older children can also cut various shapes into the halves of potatoes. Small cookie cutters are useful for sculpting these types of stamps.

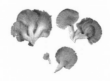

Paper Salad Collage

Materials:

- ★ Paper plates, non-toxic liquid glue or glue sticks, paint brushes or Q-tips (if using liquid glue)

- ★ Construction paper/recycled papers of various colors such as green—two or more shades of green are good, if you've got them; tear into varying-sized pieces for the lettuce/greens

- ★ Red—cut into half moons or small circles for tomatoes

- ★ Orange—cut or turn into "carrot shreds"

- ★ Brown—cut into small crouton squares, brush glue onto one side, and dip into real sesame seeds

- ★ Purple—turn into "cabbage shreds"

- ★ White—cut into thin onion rings

Older children can craft the veggies. For my preschoolers I have fun making them ahead of time for them to select from and glue onto their plates. Children who do not yet use scissors can help tear the paper, such as with the torn greens, or brush on glue and dip croutons into the sesame seeds. I recommend giving children full rights to their creativity by not making a model for them to follow or guiding their placement of the veggies. Once they know how to glue, let them decide to stack them high or simply paste a couple of pieces. (I know it's tempting to make a grown-up looking salad, but do that on your own plate.)

Seed-and-Bean Mosaics

With a mixed variety of dried beans and seeds, you can make mosaic art. Peas, red lentils, mung beans, and adzukis all lend nice color. You can also save your seeds after eating melon, cherries, or squash. Just clean them of food and set them aside for a few weeks to dry.

Materials:

- Colorful assortment of dry beans, legumes, and seeds
- Small cups or bowls
- Poster board or recycled cardboard squares (or other desired shapes)
- Glue
- Pencil

Set up a workspace by pouring each colored bean and seed in its own separate cup or bowl. Younger children gain creative confidence working free-style (not necessarily making a picture of any specific object). To make a seed-and-bean frame, cut out the middle of your cardboard square before gluing beans and seeds.

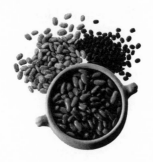

Apple-Seed Beads

Every time you eat an apple, string the seeds!

Supplies needed:

- 🌾 Fresh apple seeds (same day as the apple is eaten so they don't dry out)

- 🌾 Embroidery needle

- 🌾 Embroidery floss

- 🌾 Cutting board, cardboard scrap (or other suitable surface)

Place one apple seed on a cutting board and push a threaded needle through the center of the seed. Pull the floss through the hole and repeat with the other seeds. Allow the apple seeds to dry while strung on the floss to ensure a big enough hole. Beads can then be re-strung onto different threads in combination with other types of beads. Craft the beads into necklaces, bracelets, anklets, earrings, etc.

🌿 MINIATURE GARDENS

Eating in places with live plants in their windows is always good.

— Miss Piggy, *Miss Piggy's Guide to Life*

Even if you don't have a yard where you live, you can still have a little garden! In order to grow some types of sprouts for example, all that you need are sprouting jars, water, and a sunny spot by the window. Outdoor window boxes, micro-green flats, and patio pots are fun possibilities as well.

Growing Window Box Edibles

A box full of flowers adds grace to any window. If you've got limited garden space or simply wish for fresh ingredients near the kitchen, plant a pretty window box combining herbs and edible flowers.

Herbs and flowers to choose from: Rosemary, basil, calendula, lavender, marigold (French or signet types), nasturtium, parsley, dill, chive, marjoram, tarragon, anise hyssop, pansy, sage, lemon balm, viola, mint, and thyme. There are many other edible herbs and flowers, but some are outright poisonous. Make sure you know which is which and avoid any confusion by not planting them together in the same box. If you have young children, it is best not to keep poisonous plants in your home at all.

Growing tips: Most herbs and flowers thrive on lots of water and direct sunlight and proper drainage. If your plants have differing watering requirements, plant herbs that need less moisture (such as rosemary) in a separate pot within the box and water the flowers and herbs around it more frequently. If your window box doesn't have any drainage holes, have a grown-up drill some for you, and then cover them with coffee filters to keep the soil from running out.

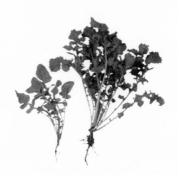

Potato Pigs

Here in Arizona we have big, wild pigs called javelenas. When they get excited the hair on their backs stands straight. Make a portly potato pig and watch its green hair grow!

Materials:

- Large yam or sweet potato with a snout-shaped end
- Spoon
- 2 whole cloves or black-eyed peas
- 2 pistachio-nut-shell halves
- 1 thick toothpick
- 4 short sticks
- Wheat berries
- Soil
- Water

To make the pig: Hollow out the potato with your spoon. Stick in the cloves or black-eyed peas for eyes and the pistachio shells for the ears. Next poke in the 4 stubby sticks on the bottom for the legs.

To plant and grow the wheat grass: Lay a 1-inch layer of soil on the bottom inside and cover with a thin layer of wheat berries. Lay another thin layer of soil on top of the wheat berries and sprinkle it all with water. Sprinkle the soil once a day to keep it moist but with not enough water to create a puddle). Within just a few days, your wheat berries will sprout.

Variation: Use a large, round, white potato instead of a yam and glue on a hollowed walnut-shell half for the snout.

Living-Food Science Experiments

Many a poignant lesson is gained by simply observing nature's ways. Conducting family experiments together is also a lot more fun then hearing (or giving) the same old spiel about just how "such-and-such food is good for you." You may wish to record your experiments in a journal, logging the various steps, observations, final results, and any concluding thoughts.

Experiment #1: Is It Living?

Take one raw carrot (that no longer has its green leaves) and one carrot that has been boiled. Cut the tops off both of the carrots, leaving about 1" of the carrot below. Set each of the carrot tops in their own bowl filled with fresh water. Label one bowl "Carrot One" and the other "Carrot Two." Place the bowls in a windowsill and leave them there for a number of days. Check the water level periodically and log any changes to the carrot tops that you observe.

Experiment #2: Is It the Same?

Grow two jars of sprouts: In jar 1, use only purified water to soak the seeds (tap water is fine for rinsing). In jar 2, use the same kind of seeds, but use only purified water that has been heated in a microwave and then allowed to cool to room temperature (use this water for the soaking and rinsing). The microwave-treated water may look, smell, taste, and feel the same as the untreated water, but is it the same?!

Experiment #3: Read Your Tongue

Objects needed:

- 🍃 Slice of sweet fruit (such as apple or banana)

- 🍃 Slice of citrus fruit (lemon, lime, orange, or grapefruit)

Take a look at the picture (right) and gently touch the different parts of your (or your child's) tongue with something citrus. You may notice that the most distinctive sensation will be received by the sour sections. Next, rinse your mouth with water and try it again with the sweet fruit. On which part of your tongue does it taste the best?

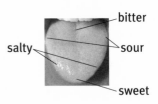

🌿 CHILDREN'S BOOK LIST

Storybooks with food, garden, and seasonal themes are invaluable resources. They set the stage for whimsical, joyful food associations, and for imaginative play. Next time you visit your local public library, make a point to dig around for one of these treasures. Here are a few that you may enjoy:

1. *The Carrot Seed* written by Ruth Kraus and illustrated by Crockett Johnson is a simple, heartwarming story about a boy who believes in a carrot seed. (I liked this one as a child.)

2. Saxton Freymann and Joost Effers have a series of picture books that feature photos of comical fruit and vegetable animals and other characters. These include: *Play with Your Food, How Are You Peeling? One Lonely Sea Horse, Gus and Button,* and *Baby Food.*

3. *Herb the Vegetarian Dragon* written by Jules Bass and illustrated by Debbie Harter is a clever story about tolerance for diverse, dietary food choices. (It is most appropriate for school-age children.)

4. *The Story of the Root Children* by Sibylle Von Olfers is a German classic with tender imagery of the natural world and the seasons.

5. *A Gardener's Alphabet* by Mary Azarian is an alphabetical walk through the garden, illustrated with wood block prints.

6. *Eating the Alphabet: Fruits and Vegetables from A to Z* by Lois Ehlert has cheery water-colored pictures of fresh fruits and veggies. It had our 1½-year-old giggling out the words "rutabaga" and "radicchio."

7. *Tops and Bottoms* by Janet Steven is a story of a lazy bear and a wily hare that share a garden together.

8. *Peter in Blueberry Land* by Elsa Beskow tells the enchanted blueberry adventure of a boy named Peter.

9. *Children of the Forest* by Elsa Beskow features themes such as seasonal changes, harvest time, and kindness toward animals.

10. The much-loved collage-art counting book *The Very Hungry Caterpillar* by Eric Carle is a good one for talking about how our bodies feel after a food-binge. The caterpillar incidentally feels much better after eating his way through a "nice green leaf."

11. *The Gigantic Turnip* by Aleksei Tolstoy and Niamh Sharkey is based on a Russian folktale about an elderly couple who grow a turnip in their garden that is so enormous they cannot uproot it without the help of some animal friends.

12. The 14 Forest Mice series by Kazuo Iwamura includes *The 14 Forest Mice and the Harvest Moon, The 14 Forest Mice and the Winter Sledding Day, The 14 Forest Mice and the Spring Meadow Picnic,* and *The 14 Forest Mice and the Summer Laundry Day.* These charming picture books feature themes of changing seasons and little forest mice by the names of Iris, Cashew, Pecan, Daisy, and Chestnut.

Part III

References, Further Reading, and Resources

❧ References

❧ Books

Benyus, Janine M. 1997. *Biomimcry: Innovation Inspired by Nature*. New York: William, Morrow and Company, Inc.

Calbom, Cherie, and Maureen Keane. 1992. *Juicing for Life*. New York: Avery Publishing.

Cousens, Gabriel. 2002. *Conscious Eating*. Berkeley, CA: North Atlantic Books.

—. 2005. *Spiritual Nutrition*. Berkeley, CA: North Atlantic Books.

Eisenberg, Eileen, Heidi Murkoff, and Sandee Hathaway. 1999. *What to Expect the First Year*. New York: Workman Publishing.

Firkaly, Susan. 1984. *Into the Mouths of Babes*. White Hall, VA: Better Way Publishers Inc.

Huggins, Kathleen. 1990. *The Nursing Mother's Companion*. Boston: Harvard Common Press.

Ildol, Olin, N.C., C.N.C. 2002. *Pregnancy, Children and the Hallelujah Diet*. Shelby, NC: Hallelujah Acres.

Jarvis, D.C., M.D. 1995. *Folk Medicine*. Fawcett.

Kendall, Francis. 1988. *Sweet Temptations*. New York: Avery Publishing.

Kitzinger, Shiela. 1998. *Breastfeeding Your Baby*. New York: Knopf Publishing.

Klaper, Michael, M.D. 1997. *Pregnancy, Children, and the Vegan Diet*. Paia, HI: Gentle World, Inc.

Martina, Roy. 1990. *Bioenergetic Nutrition*. Glendale, CA: Apex Energetics.

163

Miller, Susie, and Karen Knowler. 2000. *Feel-Good Food: A Guide to Intuitive Eating*. London: The Women's Press Ltd.

Montgomery, Beth. 2001. *Transitioning to Health*. San Diego: Nature's First Law.

Olaf, Michael. 2001. *Child of the World, Essential Montessori*. Arcata, CA: Olaf Montessori.

Patenaude, Frederick. 2002. *Sunfood Cuisine*. San Diego: Genesis Publishing.

Pennybacker, Mindy, and Aisha Ikramuddin. 1999. *Natural Baby Care*. New York: John Wiley and Sons Inc.

Pitchford, Paul. 1993. *Healing with Whole Foods*. Berkeley, CA: North Atlantic Books.

Profet, Margie. 1995. *Protecting Your Baby-to-Be*. Boston: Little Brown.

Romano, Rita. 1992. *Dining in the Raw*. New York: Kensington Publishing.

Shannon, Nomi. 1999. *The Raw Gourmet*. Burnaby, B.C., Canada: Alive Books.

Tracy, Lisa. 1989. *Kid Food*. New York: Dell Publishing Group.

Weed, Susan. 1986. *Herbal for the Childbearing Year*. Woodstock, NY: Ash Tree Publishing.

Wolfe, David. 1999. *The Sunfood Diet Success System*. San Diego: Maul Brothers Publishing.

Yaron, Ruth. 1998. *Super Baby Food*. Archibald, PA: F.J. Roberts Publishing Co.

❧ ARTICLES

Driver, Doh. 2003. "Flaxseed oil: Putting it to good use." April. www.vegfamily.com.

Institute of Bio-Terrain Sciences. "Overview of the Bio-Terrain." http://www.terrainmed.com.

KellyMom.com. 2003. "Why delay solids?" April. http://www.kellymom.com.

Margulis, Jennifer. 2002. "Mommy, I want nummies!: The benefits of nursing past three." *Mothering* magazine, November-December.

New Beginnings. 2001. "Cultural aspects of starting solids." March-April,
    Vol. 18 No. 2, 64–65.
Parenting magazine. 2004. "Deciding to go veggie." July.
Tiller, William. 1996. "Foundations of electro-dermal devices." International Congress of Electro-Dermal Screening.

❦ Further Reading

❦ HEALTH BOOKS

Bioenergetic Nutrition by Roy Martina, M.D.
Conscious Eating by Gabriel Cousens, M.D.
Enzyme Nutrition by Edward Howell
Healing Myths by Donald Epstein
Pregnancy, Children, and the Vegan Diet by Michael Klaper, M.D.
Raw Kids by Sheryl Stoycoff (one family's story of how their son's symptoms of A.D.H.D. were reversed through the introduction of a living-foods-dominant diet!)
Spiritual Fasting by Paul Bragg
Spiritual Nutrition by Gabriel Cousens, M.D.
The Children's Health Food Book by Ron Seaborn
The Mucousless Diet by Arnold Ehret
The Raw Family by Victoria Boutenko
The Sunfood Diet Success System by David Wolfe
The Tibetan Book of Living and Dying by Sogyal Rinpoche
The Twelve Stages of Healing by Donald Epstein
The Vegan Sourcebook by Joanne Stepaniak
Vegan Nutrition, Pure and Simple by Michael Klaper, M.D.

❧ Recipe Books

Angel Foods by Cherie Soria
Dining in the Raw by Rita Romano (combines living foods with macrobiotic cooking techniques)
Eat Smart Eat Raw by Kate Wood
Hooked on Raw by Rhio
Living on Live Food by Alissa Cohen
Raw: The Uncook Book by Juliano Brotman and Erika Lenkert
Sunfood Cuisine by Frederic Patenaude
Sweet Temptations by Francis Kendall
The Raw Gourmet by Nomi Shannon
Vital Creations by Chad Sarno
Warming Up to Living Foods by Elisa Markowitz

❧ Practitioners and Testing

Association for Network Chiropractic
444 Main Street
Longmont, CO 80501
303-678-8101 • www.associationfornetworkcare.com

Bioenergetic Testing and Futureplex Homeoenergetic Remedies
Apex Energetics
1701 E. Edinger Ave. #A-4
Santa Ana, CA 92705
714-973-7733 • www.apexenergetics.com

Contact Reflex Analysis Foundation
P.O. Box 87413
Vancouver, WA 98687-7413
360-882-8177 • www.crahealth.org

A personalized system of health evaluation testing the body with its own bioelectricity.

Matrix Nutritional Consulting
P.O. Box 203
Gays Mills, WI 54631
www.babygreensbooks.com
Comprehensive individual nutrition, health plans, and educational support.

Terrain Testing
Institute of Bio-Terrain Sciences
866-204-9026 • www.terrainmed.com

Tree of Life Foundation and Retreat Center
Patagonia, AZ 85624

❦ BREASTFEEDING/MILK

Human Milk Banking Association of North America (HMBANA)
8 Jan Sebastian Way, #13
Sandwich, MA 02563
888-232-8809 or 508-888-4041
Fax: 508-888-8050

La Leche League International (Breastfeeding support organization)
www.lalecheleague.org

❦ GOODS AND INFORMATION

The Fresh Network
P.O. Box 71
Ely
Camps
CB6 32Q UK
Tel: +44(0)-870-800-7070 • Info@fresh-network.com

Living Nutrition **magazine**
>P.O. Box 256
>Sebastopol, CA 95473
>www.livingnutrition.com

Nature's First Law
>P.O. Box 900202
>San Diego, CA 95473
>www.rawfood.com

North American Vegetarian Society
>www.navs-online.org

✤ Bulk Organic Foods

✤ SPROUTING

Kid's Sprout Exploration Kit:

The Sproutpeople
>225 Main Street
>Gays Mills, WI 54631
>www.sproutpeople.com

Large selection of sprouting seeds and supplies.

The Sprout House
>P.O. Box 754131
>Forest Hills, NY 11375
>www.sprouthouse.com

Sun Organic Farm
>Box 2429
>Valley Center, CA 92082
>1-888-269-9888

Resource for organic seeds for sprouting and greens.

❧ WHEAT GRASS

Green Pastures Wheatgrass
1035 Parkway Industrial Park Drive #104
Buford, GA 30518
www.greenpastureswheatgrass.com

Greenward Nurseries and New Native Sprouts
P.O. Box 1413
Freedom, CA 95019
408-728-4136
Source for certified organic wheatgrass and sprouts.

Wheatgrass Direct
P.O. Box 249
Ottsville, PA 18942
1-877-5JUICED • www.wheatgrassdirect.com
*Home delivery of certified organic wheatgrass and 25 varieties
of sprouts.*

❧ ONLINE RESOURCES

www.babygreensbooks.com (private and group consultations and classes,
   teleseminars)
www.borntolove.com (extensive line of baby/kid supplies, toys, etc.)
www.diaperfabric.com (patterns and sewing supplies for make-it-yourself
   diapers and clothing; hemp and other fabrics at wholesale prices)
www.brainchildmag.com (the magazine for thinking mothers)
www.fresh-network.com (large, raw-foods site based in the U.K.)
www.gourmetgreens.com (shipper and grower of fresh wheat grass and
   soil-grown salad greens)
www.hipmama.com (alternative parenting site)
www.livingright.com (lowest-price guarantees on best-selling kitchen
   appliances)

www.nomorefakenews.com (well-researched articles on the underre-
ported dark side of medicine and other subjects—often with a slant
toward the effects on kids)
www.rawchef.org (online home of Vital Creations chef services, raw
foods artistry, and resources)
www.sprouthouse.com (organic seeds for sprouting)
www.sproutman.com (comprehensive resource for all sprouting needs)
www.vegetarianbaby.com (comprehensive resource for the vegetarian
baby and child)

✤ Open-pollinated and Heirloom Garden Seeds

Pinetree Garden Seeds
P.O. Box 300
New Gloucester, ME 04260
207-926-3400

Seeds of Change
P.O. Box 15700
Santa Fe, NM 87506
888-762-7333 • www,seedsofchange.com

Seed Savers Exchange
3076 North Winn Rd.
Decorah, IA 52101
www.seedsaver.com

✤ Organic Cold-pressed Oils

Adam's Olive Ranch
19401 Road 220
Strathmore, CA 93267
888-216-5483

Barleans Organic Oils

4936 Lake Terrell Road
Ferndale, WA 98248
460-380-6367 • www.barleans.com

Omega Nutrition U.S.A.

6515 Aldrich Road
Bellingham, WA 98226
800-661-FLAX • www.omegaflo.com

Sun Organic Farms

Box 2429
Valley Center, CA 92082
888-269-9888 • www.sunorganic.com

☙ DRIED FOODS

Azure Standard

79709 Dufar Valley Road
Dufar, OR 97021
541-467-2230 • www.azurefarm.com

Source for quality bulk foods.

Eden Foods

701 Tecumseh Road
Clinton, MI 49236
517-456-7424 • www.edenfoods.com

Living Tree Community Foods

P.O. Box 10082
Berkeley, CA 94709
510-420-1440 • www.livingtreecommunity.com

Sun Organic Farms

Box 2429
Valley Center, CA 92082
888-269-9888 • www.sunorganic.com

Large selection of high quality organic foods.

✿ SEA VEGETABLES AND MISO

Goldmine Natural Foods

7805 Arjons Drive
San Diego, CA 92126
800-475-3663 • www.goldminenaturalfoods.com

✿ SEA VEGETABLES, CELTIC SEA SALT, AND GRAINS

Maine Coast Sea Vegetables

Box 78
Franklin, ME 04634
237-565-2907 • www.seaveg.com

High quality sea vegetables, strict quality control, and testing for toxins.

Mendocino Sea Vegetable Company

P.O. Box 1265
Mendocino, CA 95460
707-937-2050 • www.seaweed.net

South River Miso Inc.

South River Farm
Conway, MA 01341

Live organic miso.

✿ ORGANIC PRODUCE DELIVERY

Eco Organics of New Jersey

201-333-8840 • www.eco-organics.com

Diamond Organics

P.O. Box 2159
Freedom, CA 95019
888-ORGANIC • www.diamondorganics.com

Pikarco

P.O. Box 924095
Homestead, FL 33092
305-247-8650 • www.pikarco.com

Veritable Vegetables

1100 Cesar Chavez Street
San Francisco, CA 94124
415-641-3500

❧ SNACKS

Natureraw

P.O. Box 18
Fulton, CA 95439
707-527-7959 • www.natureraw.com

Organic crackers and desserts.

Nature's High Unique Foods

P.O. Box 19495
Boulder, CO 80308
303-545-2145 • www.natureshighuniquefoods.com

Prepared foods made from raw dried foods.

Snacks Alive

560-B Mystery Spot Road
Santa Cruz, CA 95065
831-423-0226

Low-temperature dried candies, crackers, and desserts.

❦ Tools and Equipment

www.discountjuicers.com

Good source for juicers and dehydrators.

Excalibur Dehydrator
68083 Power Inn Road
Sacramento, CA 95824
916-381-4254

Green Power Juicer
Downey, CA 90241
888-254-7336 • www.greenpower.com

Health Force Regeneration Systems
P.O. Box 5005
Rancho Santa Fe, CA 92067
800-537-2717 • www.healthforce.net

Plastaket Manufacturing
6220 E. Hwy. 12
Lodi, CA 95240
209-369-2154 • www.championjuicer.com

Vita-Mix Corp.
8615 Usher Road
Cleveland, OH 44138
800-848-2649 • www.vitamix.com

❦ WATER IONIZERS

The Water Cats
e-mail: jaku_ma@yahoo.com
www.babygreensbooks.com